# Weight a Minute!

## Transform Your Health in 60 Seconds a Day

### Deborah Enos, CN
#### The One-Minute Wellness Coach

4 grams of sugar = 1 teaspoon
1 packet of sugar = 1 teaspoon

10 9 8 7 6 5 4 3 2

Printed in the United States of America

LCCN 2007920226

ISBN 978-0-9820219-0-3

Editor: Debby Nagusky

Cover Design: Jef Serio

Cover Photograph: Vince Vonada, V2 Photography

Interior Layout: Stephanie Martindale

Proofreader: Julie Scandora

# Contents

Transform Your Health
in 60 Seconds a Day

Transform Your Health
in 60 Seconds a Day

# Acknowledgments

Writing this book was truly a labor of love on the part of many people in my life. I've been working on this book for eight months—well, actually, eight months plus seven years of failed attempts!

First and foremost, I thank God for the guidance, wisdom and, most of all, the grace in putting this book together.

Thank you to my sweet, patient, loving and gorgeous husband, Steve, who never got frustrated with my time spent away from him and who patiently smiled through the late dinners and piles of unfolded laundry. You have supported me through every aspect of this book. I'm so happy to be married to my best friend.

To my darling and fun girls, Jordan and Alexandra. You were so sweet about asking me how many pages I had written before you would allow me into the summer badminton games. If I missed my writing goal you graciously sent me back to my office to finish. Thank you, girls, for your love and devotion. I love watching you both grow up as confident and content young women of God.

Thank you to my wonderful and loving parents. You two have always supported me in every aspect of my life. I am who I am because of you.

Thank you to all of my clients from 1988 through today. You have inspired me to write a book for those yearning to feel better but who are too tired, busy and worn-out to spend hours researching solutions to their health problems.

To my brilliant and creative editor, Debby Nagusky. You truly have gotten inside my head and made my words so much more interesting and compelling. You were a dream to work with.

Thank you so much to Jef Serio of Serious Design for his creative cover and book title.

Transform Your Health
in 60 Seconds a Day

# About the author

It was 1996, and I'd been working in the wellness field for eight years. On this particular Monday morning, I was seeing my client Mary. Mary had hired me to help her get her body and diet into tiptop shape. She was in her early 60s, recently widowed and ready to take on her new life with energy and enthusiasm. She had responded positively to all my suggestions regarding exercise and dietary changes I believed she needed to make to optimize her health and energy. At the end of our session she asked me if she could show me something. Great, I thought, she has a new recipe or a new pair of the latest and greatest power-walking shoes. Of course I told her I wanted to see what she had to show me.

"Wonderful!" she said as she placed her hand on my arm and walked me over to her full-length mirror. She reached out and grabbed a pointer from the shelf behind me and then proceeded to point out and circle with her pointer all the areas on my body that she felt needed liposuction.

Hmmm … this wasn't quite what I was expecting.

Mary told me she felt I needed to see my faults for two reasons:

1. No one can feel inspired by an overweight trainer and nutritionist.

2. I was going to drive away any potential clients because I was so chubby.

It's true, I *was* an overweight trainer and nutritionist, and I was eating for all the wrong reasons. I was working two jobs and was in a deeply troubling relationship. I had nearly debilitating back pain, high cholesterol, asthma, anxiety disorder and insomnia. I certainly wasn't the picture of health, with exhaustion being one of the most troubling aspects of my life at this time. I was choosing unhealthy foods and sugary caffeinated drinks as quick pick-me-ups just to get through the next appointment, and then I would crash and choose another unhealthy food as a boost to get me through the next couple of hours. I was only 31 but felt old, tired and defeated.

While I didn't appreciate the way my client broached the topic, she did make it clear that it was time for me to finally deal with my own health with the same passion and purpose I was directing toward my clients' health.

During my college training in health science, I was never taught how and what to eat to increase energy, health and vitality. I learned the basic four food groups and how to help those who have diseases such as heart disease or diabetes. Disease avoidance or eating for energy wasn't part of the curriculum. I soon realized I had a lot of learning to do and began studying with a vengeance how to use food as a drug, a drug to increase energy, say, or help diffuse anxiety so you can relax and fall asleep. I began to practice my new methods, doing exactly what I needed to eat to stay alert, sharp and high-energy all day. In 12 months I lost 40 pounds, regained my energy and lowered my cholesterol to well under 200. My back pain was almost gone, and I was off all of my medications for anxiety, insomnia and asthma. I was no longer sick and tired, and my moods were steady. I felt good, and I continue to feel great each day.

# About this book

When feeling overwhelmed, busy and exhausted, the last thing you want to do is sit down with a 300-page nutrition textbook and figure out how to help yourself. I've done that for you by reading thousands of pages of research and filtering down the essentials into bite-size chunks that are easy to apply to your life immediately. Each chapter uses a "**What-Why-How**" approach to specific health issues (**what** is the problem, **why** is it a problem, and **how** can you fix it), and each can be read in a minute or less. Finally, a nutrition book that is a quick read and easy to digest!

Keep this book handy—in your car, desk or briefcase—so it's there when you need to make choices, such as picking the healthiest fast foods (when fast food is the only food), or what to snack on to increase your mental sharpness, or how to boost your immune system to protect against disease.

As we all get busier, we look for shortcuts. This is a book of extensively and carefully researched shortcuts. I hope it helps you attain the level of health and energy you strive for.

# Section 1:
# Dieting, Eating Habits
# and Weight Loss

# Section 1:
# Dieting, Eating Habits and Weight Loss

I was sitting down with my new client, Emily, who was telling me about her battles with weight loss: "I've struggled my whole life; even as a little girl I had to wear pants from the 'husky' clothing section. I did okay through college, but once I graduated I slowly started to gain, about five to eight pounds a year. Now I have a 5-year-old, and I'm still telling people I just had a baby! I don't eat that much during the day; in fact, I often skip lunch so I can leave work a little early. Now I'm finding that I'm relying more on caffeine and diet soda to get me through my afternoon slump. I feel tired and grumpy most of the day, even on my days off! It seems as I get older my metabolism is getting slower and slower, and if I just look at a cookie, I'll gain a pound."

Is your story anything like Emily's?

Emily's health goals are to lose weight and maintain the loss, increase her energy, and create a food plan that will help her keep her mood and energy steady all day. Her current pattern of eating a small, or no, breakfast, often skipping lunch and then eating a Thanksgiving-size meal for dinner, combined with some stress, will only lead to continued weight gain.

Transform Your Health
in 60 Seconds a Day

To reach her goals, I advised Emily to make these changes to her daily routine:

 Always eat a high-energy breakfast. This meal should be large enough to keep you full for at least three hours. Include protein here to keep you fuller and more alert through the morning.

 Always eat lunch! Skipping it will set you up to be starving all afternoon, which will make you give into your sugar cravings, which will cause the afternoon doldrums to hit, which will make you want to take a nap.

 Make dinner the smallest meal of the day. If you eat a substantial mid-afternoon snack you won't be as hungry at dinner.

# Increase your food,
# decrease your waistline

## WHAT:

You're eating a lot less and still can't lose weight. You are beginning to wonder how you can possibly cut back more. This approach is ineffective. The more you reduce your calories, the more you turn down your metabolism. The lower your metabolism, the less fat and calories you burn.

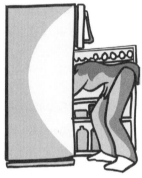

## WHY:

Here's how it works: The body gets used to functioning on a certain number of calories daily, let's say 1,500. If you reduce that number by a small amount, say 300, you will lose some weight. But if you continue to lower your caloric intake (instead of increasing exercise) your body will go into starvation mode and try to protect itself by burning very little fat and slowing down your metabolic rate. Your body, especially a woman's body, likes to have extra fat, just in case there is a famine around the corner.

# HOW:

 Cut back on a small amount of calories while increasing your exercise. The exercise will add muscle to your body, and more muscle will increase your metabolism so that you will be a fat-burning machine all day long. You will burn more calories while you sleep, eat, work and play.

 Eat all day. Spreading your calories throughout the day prompts your body to burn more calories. Every time you eat, you raise your body temperature, which is, in essence, your metabolism. People who eat five to six times per day burn more calories and lose more weight than people who eat only one or two meals a day.

 Eat the majority of your calories during the day, when you need the most energy. If your biggest meal of the day is right before bed, your body has no opportunity to burn off those calories through activity.

 Eat within a half-hour of getting up. Your metabolism sleeps while you sleep. It needs a little food to wake it up in the morning. As soon as you eat, it reports to work and starts burning fat and calories. It doesn't take a huge breakfast to turn on your metabolism. If you're not hungry in the morning, start your day with a hundred-calorie snack—a piece of fruit or a glass of milk.

# Eat to fill and thrill!

## WHAT:

While losing weight, you need to focus on eating foods that are not only healthy but will also fill you up, satisfy you and keep you from craving foods you're trying to avoid. The more satisfied you feel, the less you will go searching for the candy bowl.

## WHY:

What are the first foods that come to mind when you think about dieting? Salads, fruit, rice cakes and water, lots of water, right? But do any of these really satisfy your appetite? Not a chance! While eating a large plate of steamed veggies is great for your health, it doesn't make much of a dent in your appetite.

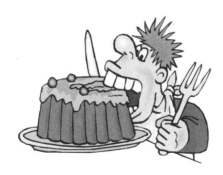

Transform Your Health
in 60 Seconds a Day

# HOW:

Dare I say it: Eat FAT!

Would it surprise you to learn that **peanuts** could be good for weight loss? The latest research shows that people who eat them are more successful at both losing weight and keeping it off. In a Harvard study looking at two groups of dieters (Mattes and Voisard 1998), the first group included an ounce of heart-healthy peanuts, peanut butter or mixed nuts once a day. The other group did not get the heart-healthy daily snack. A year and a half later the peanut group had lost the most weight and kept it off, while the non-peanut snackers had gained back 5 pounds. The researchers reasoned that the fat in peanuts kept the snackers fuller longer, thus staving off food cravings for as long as two hours when compared to other snacks. Similar findings have surfaced for olive oil, another heart-healthy fat. Dieters who included it in their diet also stayed fuller longer and avoided unhealthy snacks (Chiavacci, 2002). Don't forget that, although this oil is good for you, a little, at 100 calories per tablespoon, goes a long way.

Here are some simple food combos that can keep you fuller longer:

 Add a tablespoon of peanut butter to an apple.

 Sprinkle a tablespoon of olive oil on steamed veggies, or sauté veggies in a tablespoon of it.

 Eat a small handful of trail mix with your non-fat latté.

 Add a small can of tuna or salmon to your green salad.

# Are you a fat-burning machine or a fat-making machine?

### WHAT:

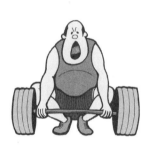

The world is divided into two types of people, those who can eat anything they want and still maintain their weight, and those who look at a piece of cake and gain weight. The former burn up calories and fat as fast as they eat them, and the latter store those calories as fat for the winter, 12 months a year.

### WHY:

Some people are born with a high metabolism, but it is possible to rev up slow metabolism and turn your body into a fat-burning machine.

## HOW:

There are two keys to turning your body into a fat-burning machine:

1.  Add more muscle to your body. One pound of muscle burns approximately 80 calories a day. One pound of fat burns only two calories a day. Choose exercises that will add muscle to your frame to increase your daily calorie burn.

2.  Burn calories, don't cut them. People who have lost weight and kept it off know the importance of staying active. In fact, a recent study on fidgeting shows that multiple movements throughout the day can play a tremendous role in weight loss and weight-loss maintenance (Levine and Eberhardt 1999). Many people in

Transform Your Health
in 60 Seconds a Day

the study moved enough to burn an extra 850 calories a day, the equivalent of an 8.5-mile walk!

Here are a few ways to add muscle to your body and increase calories burned:

 Take the stairs. An extra 10 minutes of stair climbing a day will burn 12 pounds of fat a year.

 Do standing push-ups against your kitchen or bathroom counter.

 Do lunges or squats while on the phone or watching TV.

 Work in the garden.

 Actively play (lifting and moving) with kids.

 Walk more. An extra 10 minutes of walking each day will burn almost 5 pounds of fat a year. It really does pay to park your car in the farthest space from the store!

 Link your house chores into one long cardio segment. Start your day by raking leaves, then wash the car and walk the dog. These activities could add up to an hour or more of fat burning.

 Throw away your remote control and actually walk over to the TV to change channels.

 Just move. Any activity is better than no activity.

# Mini-meals, maxi-health

## WHAT:

You wake up late, grab coffee and run out the door. It's now 2 p.m., your energy is gone and you're starving. Someone in the office suggests ordering a pizza so you can all keep on working. Three inhaled pieces of triple-cheese-pepperoni later, you're tired, cranky and ready for a nap.

## WHY:

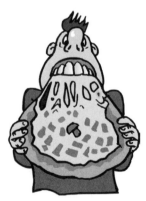

When you skip meals, your blood sugar drops dramatically. When your blood sugar drops, you drop, and you lose your productivity, focus and energy. Then you eat too much, trying to fill the hole in your gut, and afterwards all you can think about is taking a nap, since overeating is a message to your body to sleep.

Transform Your Health
in 60 Seconds a Day

# HOW:

Snack, snack, snack! The most effective and efficient people I know eat at least two snacks per day along with three smaller meals. Many of these people even snack before a meal!

If you don't feel ravenous at breakfast, forget the big breakfast and have a snack. You might eat an apple upon rising and then at work have a bowl of oatmeal with some nuts added in.

Forget the old adage: "A snack will ruin your appetite." A healthy snack will help us avoid foods that aren't energy-producing and will keep us from overeating.

Always have a snack ready. Keep a small packet of trail mix, a piece of fruit or a meal-replacement bar handy for emergencies.

Change your mindset. I'm giving you permission to eat many mini-meals all day long.

# The after-dinner danger zone

## WHAT:

Many of us usually blow it after dinner by trying to avoid eating something sweet. We may sample four or five different foods before we finally succumb to the cookies. If we had just gone for the cookies right away, we would have eaten fewer calories on the way to finding them.

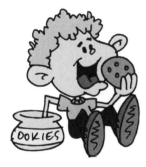

## WHY ...
## ...do you crave something sweet after a meal?

Some nutritionists say it's because your body is trying to balance out all the salt you just consumed. By eating something sweet, you bring your body back into balance. In a way this makes sense, or am I the only one who has chased a bowl of salty popcorn with a scoop of ice cream?

Transform Your Health
in 60 Seconds a Day

# HOW...
# ...to handle your sweet cravings:

Try eating fruit first. There are a few times each day when we crave a sweet. Your body often doesn't even care *what* it is as long as it's sweet because it's looking for a quick "wake-up," and the fastest way to wake it up is by eating something sweet.

So next time you're craving something sweet, grab a tangerine or any sweet, *juicy*, fruit (non-juicy bananas aren't the best choice). Eat the tangerine and wait five minutes for the fruit sugar to hit your bloodstream and give your body the sugar boost it was craving. After five minutes, if you still want the cookie, you can have it, but because you've already had a small sugar hit from the fruit, your body won't need as many cookies. Many of my clients and I find that after eating the fruit, we no longer have any desire for the cookies.

This really does work, but you must be prepared to grab something healthy first, so keep the fruit right on your desk and the cookies out of reach. If you have to get up and get the fruit you probably won't do it, but most of us would happily walk a mile for some really good cookies!

A few other ideas to kill your after-meal sugar cravings:

- Brush your teeth. This will completely change your focus and usually kills your desire for something sweet.

- Drink a cup of tea or low-calorie hot chocolate.

- Chew some gum or suck on a piece of hard candy.

# How big is your bagel?

## WHAT:

You stop at the bagel place on your way to work, pick up your favorite kind and chow it down in the car. At lunch, your office sends out for sandwiches, and then you pop a bag of popcorn for your mid-afternoon snack. Would you believe that by the time you'd finished your bagel you had hit the 50 percent mark for you daily bread carbs, and by the end of the day you'd had a two-day supply of carbs?

## WHY:

Over-portioning has been a "growing" movement for the last 20 years. Food manufacturers have been slowly increasing the serving sizes of our food, so slowly that most people don't remember that the original serving size for a soda was approximately 6 ounces, compared to approximately 16 ounces today, or 6, versus 16, teaspoons of sugar.

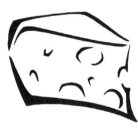

The problem is we have no idea what a real serving looks like. Did you know that most restaurant pasta dishes contain enough for two, if not three, people? Most also pack a whopping 1,000-plus calories after the addition of Parmesan cheese.

 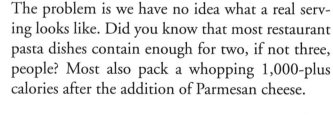

Here are guidelines to help you gauge appropriate amounts of some foods:

 **Pastas, grains and cereals**

¾ cup—a little bigger than a tennis ball

 **Meat, fish and poultry**

3 ounces—about the size of a deck of cards

 **Nuts**

1 ounce—the size of a shot glass, will just cover the palm of your hand

 **Vegetables and fruits**

One cup is a serving, but these can be eaten in almost unlimited amounts. One cup is about the size of your fist.

# NEWSFLASH: Studies show it's easy to gain weight as we age.

Wow. That's a real shocker.

### WHAT:

It's amazing how easy it is to gain weight as we age—it seems to happen so quickly. On average, we eat 300 more calories daily than we did 30 years ago, and we weigh 30 pounds more than we did 30 years ago. Coincidence? I don't think so.

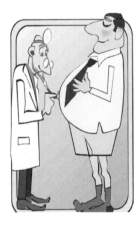

### WHY:

We gain weight when we eat 100 more calories a day than our body can burn. And those 100 calories are so easy to eat. Some examples:

- Adding an extra pat of butter

- Eating just five bites of mac' n' cheese

- Switching from a small to a large latté

- Eating the small bag of chips that comes with your sandwich

But it's not just the food. Take a look at how few calories you burn living your cushy lifestyle:

- Grabbing the closest parking space costs you 40 calories a day, or almost 5 pounds of fat gained a year.

Transform Your Health
in 60 Seconds a Day

- Taking the elevator instead of the stairs costs you 50 calories a day, or over 5 pounds of fat gained a year.

- E-mailing messages instead of walking over to talk to someone costs you 60 calories per day, or over 6 pounds of fat gained a year.

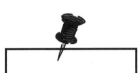

You could gain 16 pounds of fat a year from all of these habits.

# HOW...

## ...can you ward off the weight gain that comes with aging?

 Add in movement to your day by always taking the stairs and parking far away from your destination.

 Buy a pedometer and wear it all day. Your goal is 10,000 steps per day (5 miles)

 Don't clean up the dinner plates by eating what's left on them!

# Are you eating just for sport?

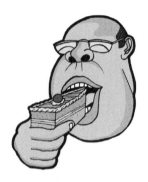

## WHAT:

Have you ever eaten when you weren't hungry? You're in good company, as recent research shows that about 50 percent of us turn to food when we're bored, lonely or really stressed out. Obviously, this is not a healthy approach to eating. In fact, researchers discovered that emotional eaters didn't feel satisfied after eating and usually felt more stress or guilt after eating for the wrong reasons (BBC News August 23, 2004).

## WHY:

Emotional eaters come in all shapes, sizes, ages and gender, but the fastest-growing group is women between the ages of 35 and 55. These women are typically high-achieving, organized and successful in most areas of their lives. (Sound like anyone you know?) The stress of overwork can make eating seem like a simple method of stress management.

Transform Your Health
in 60 Seconds a Day

# HOW...
## ... do you break this habit of reaching for food when you're not really hungry?

The simple solution is to do something else for at least two minutes. This is enough time for most of us to allow the craving to pass—unrequited of course!

**Here are a few other ideas to help curtail emotional eating:**

Drink a glass of water or try a hot beverage. Most of my clients report that after consuming a hot liquid, they just don't feel the same food cravings. By the way, a hot beverage is a cup of tea or water processed decaf coffee, not a triple mocha with whipped cream!

Go outside. A change of scene, even for a minute or two, can change our endorphin levels. You will feel better since you have more "happy hormones" circulating, and perhaps it will be easier not to grab the candy bar.

If you need to eat something, eat fruit! Fruit is high in fiber and water; and this dynamic duo will fill you up and make it tough to keep eating.

# Good for your budget but bad for your thighs

## WHAT:

You can order the extra-large bucket of popcorn for only 75 cents more. So now the consumer dilemma: Spend a few more pennies and get twice as much popcorn, or stick with your original choice? Your mind is telling you: "Go for the big bucket, it's a deal!" but at the same time you know how tight your jeans feel. You make the "smart-consumer" decision and go for the super-size, telling yourself you are going to eat just half of it. But two hours later the movie is over and the popcorn is gone. What happened?

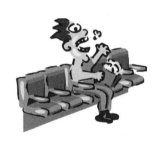

## WHY:

First of all, we know that when food is placed in front of us we eat it, all of it. And, when eating with other people, we have a tendency to eat about 30 percent more calories.

Fifty years ago you could order a fast-food meal of a burger, fries and a Coke and walk away with about a 600-calorie meal. Today that same meal will cost you about 1,500 calories. It takes an extra 3,500 calories to add a pound of fat to your body. If you eat three of these meals, you will have all the calories you need to add that pound of fat to your body.

Transform Your Health
in 60 Seconds a Day

# HOW...

## ... else do we pay the price for super-sizing?

 Fast-food burger: For an extra $1.50 we get a larger burger and more fries. Calorie cost? About 700.

 Submarine sandwich: For an extra $1.50 you can double the size of your sandwich. Calorie cost? About 500.

 Movie theater: For an extra 75 cents you can get twice as much popcorn. Calorie cost? About 500.

 Soft drinks: For less than 50 cents you can go from Big Gulp to Super Big Gulp. Calorie cost? 450.

# Sugar: friend or foe?

## WHAT:

Most Americans eat more than 150 pounds of sugar a year. To consume this much, you would have to eat a teaspoon of it 20 out of 24 hours each day, seven days a week, 52 weeks a year.

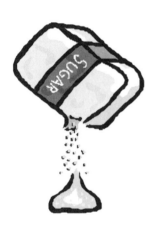

It's easy to quickly rack up the sugar points by starting with a sugary breakfast cereal (5–6 teaspoons of sugar) or jam (2–3 teaspoons) on your toast. Mid-morning you may have a pastry or muffin (8–9 teaspoons) and then have a can of soda (10–12 teaspoons) with lunch. At this point your body will crave more sugar to try and make you feel better, and the cycle continues. This is because sugar enters and exits your bloodstream quickly, causing a short-lived high followed by a crash in energy. After you crash, you will need more sugar to get the same amount of energy you got from the first "hit." By the time you get home from work, you are starving, cranky and not at your best for a peaceful evening with family or friends, or even yourself!

# WHY...
## ... sugar is a problem*:

Sugar intake is linked to type 2 diabetes, heart disease, high blood pressure, anxiety, hyperactivity, tooth decay, arthritis, eczema, sinus congestion, indigestion, obesity and giant mood swings. Sugar is also the preferred fuel for cancer-cell growth.

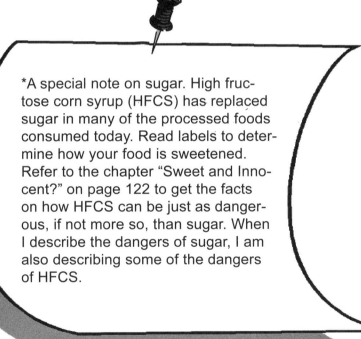

*A special note on sugar. High fructose corn syrup (HFCS) has replaced sugar in many of the processed foods consumed today. Read labels to determine how your food is sweetened. Refer to the chapter "Sweet and Innocent?" on page 122 to get the facts on how HFCS can be just as dangerous, if not more so, than sugar. When I describe the dangers of sugar, I am also describing some of the dangers of HFCS.

# HOW to curb your sugar intake:

First, determine how much sugar you and your family are ingesting each day by reading food labels. Divide the grams of sugar by 4 to determine teaspoons per servings. Remember that your limit of sugar for the day is 18 teaspoons (12–15 for your kids), and not all at once.

 Start your day with a non-sweet breakfast that includes some lean protein (eggs or lean chicken sausage) and whole grains.

 Include a lean protein at lunch.

 Drink lots of herbal tea, especially green tea. Green tea helps prevent sugar cravings by stabilizing blood sugar. See "Green tea gets the green light" on page 126 for more about the benefits of green tea.

 Eat lots of green veggies (broccoli, cabbage, asparagus and bok choy). Green veggies have a lot of magnesium, just like sugary chocolate, so eating more magnesium-rich sugar-free foods can keep chocolate cravings at bay.

 Cut your soda consumption in half.

 Avoid sugary "juice" drinks. Eat the fruit and skip the juice.

 Drink more water, sparkling or plain.

 Know the many names for sugar: high fructose corn syrup, dextrose, maltose, lactose, fructose, malt sugar and honey (this is just a partial list).

Transform Your Health
in 60 Seconds a Day

# Calorie savers to help you fit into your summer clothes any time of year

## WHAT:

Most of us gain a few pounds during the winter. Shorter days and less activity make this happen quite easily. All it takes is an extra 100 calories a day, and next thing you know you've added 10 pounds of fat to your frame in a year.

## WHY:

The key to losing that winter weight is to get rid of it as soon as you notice it. A concept in exercise science states that the older the fat, the harder it is to lose. I have seen this in my clients, especially the ones who gain weight on a cruise. Those who concentrate on losing the weight right after returning usually get rid of it quickly. The ones who wait a few months really seem to struggle with the weight loss.

# HOW...

## ... to avoid winter (or any-time-of-year) weight gain:

Limit your food choices by type and color—the more choices you have, the more you'll eat. If you're trying to cut back on your evening meal, stick with one or two food options and foods that are the same color (boring, but worth a try).

Take a paper napkin and dab the surface fat off the top of your pizza—you will save about 45 fat calories per slice. I know that doesn't seem like much, but multiply that by two pieces, 50 weeks a year (that's less pizza consumed than the national average), and you just saved yourself over a pound of fat that would have otherwise been stored just where you didn't want it!

If you order fried food, order french fries instead of onion rings and save between 200 and 1,000 calories. Let's say you save about 300 calories, times 12 servings per year—you've avoided adding a pound of fat to your body.

Remove half the meat filling from your sandwich (which usually has 2–3 protein servings on average) and save about 200 calories, depending on the type of meat. Now multiply that by two sandwiches a week for 50 weeks, and your net savings is almost 6 pounds of fat.

Transform Your Health
in 60 Seconds a Day

Drink alcohol in moderation. Alcohol is a relaxant, and studies have shown that you may eat up to 30 percent more calories during a meal because you are so "relaxed."

 Don't eat in the dark! Eating your meal with soft lighting or in the dark, like a movie theater, can cause you to eat significantly more calories.

 Get enough sleep. Find out why in the Energy and Sleep section.

 Eat an apple before lunch and dinner. (See "An apple a day" on page 56.)

 Avoid processed foods. They are low in fiber, and the less fiber you eat, the more fat you store on your body.

# The only food plan you'll ever need

### WHAT:

Learn to eat for energy and health, and if you need to lose weight, it will happen, slowly but permanently.

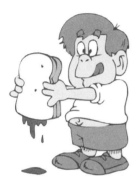

### WHY:

If you have more energy you'll be more active. People who are active are leaner and healthier than people who are more sedentary—simple, huh?

## HOW:

**EAT BREAKFAST.** Never skip this meal! Breakfast eaters burn an extra 55,000 calories a year. That's like burning an extra 15 pounds just by eating more. Always include some fat, protein and carbs at this meal. This combination of foods will keep you fuller longer and rev up your fat-burning engine for the day.

Examples:

 Hot cereal with soymilk or 1-percent milk and a small handful of nuts

Transform Your Health
in 60 Seconds a Day

One or two eggs, toast and fruit

 Veggie omelet and fruit

 Beans, eggs and low-fat cheese in a high-fiber tortilla

 Protein drink with added fiber

**SNACK.** Include a mid-morning snack to take the edge off of your hunger before lunch. This snack doesn't have to be big. If you skipped your morning fruit, have it now. If you need to boost your energy, have a fruit-protein-carb combo.

Examples:

 Apple, 1 tablespoon peanut butter and crackers

 Half a protein bar and piece of fruit

 Leftover breakfast protein drink and some crackers

 Piece of fruit and a hard-boiled egg

 One or two slices of lunch meat and a piece of fruit

**LUNCH.** The biggest meal of the day. By the end of this meal you should have eaten 50–60 percent of your day's calories.

Examples:

 Sushi: Edamame (fresh soybeans), miso soup, four to six pieces of sushi.

 Thai: Sautéed veggie and lean meat dish, any soup that is non-dairy-based. Skip the salad and Thai tea.

 Mexican: Chicken fajitas. Skip the sour cream and cheese, but have 1–2 tablespoons of guacamole.

 Lunch from home: Be creative with what's already in your fridge—leftover salad with chopped lean meat, beans or tuna on top; left-over veggie stir-fry with chicken.

**AFTERNOON SNACK.** You should be hungry three to four hours after lunch. You need a snack here so you don't eat a huge dinner. Also, if you are planning a pre-dinner workout, a snack here is imperative for good workout energy. See snack ideas above.

**DINNER.** The smallest meal of the day. If your body requires 500 calories at dinner and you give it 800, the extra 300 will be converted to fat and stored in exactly the places you don't want it. Your dinner can be a smaller version of your lunch.

To satisfy your after-dinner sweet tooth, try a cup of low-calorie hot chocolate. It will take a half-hour to drink, and by the time you finish it, your cravings should be gone. See "The after-dinner danger zone" on page 12 for more ideas to curb your sweet tooth.

# Section 2:
# Energy and Sleep

# Section 2: Energy and Sleep

Sam is a hardworking guy, always on the go. He gets up early and is answering e-mails by 7 a.m. He gets a lot accomplished before noon, which is a good thing since he loses most of his concentration, energy and motivation by early afternoon.

Most of us spend more time caring for our cars than we do our bodies. Would you drive your car to work if your gas gauge was on empty? You might make it a block or two, then it would sputter and die. This is what's happening to Sam—he never fills up his "tank" (his body). He goes as long as he can without fuel and then just stops. The simple solution here is to eat and drink well first thing in the morning. In fact, what you consume then can affect what you crave in the afternoon. Starting your day with a little bit of animal protein will make you crave sugar less and reduce your appetite overall.

Eating and drinking for peak performance and getting adequate sleep are things many of us are not doing.

Sam requested a program from me that will help increase his afternoon energy and focus. He would also like to have enough zip for a trip to the gym or a jog after work.

Here's part of the program I designed for Sam. It may work for you too:

1. Avoid sugary drinks, juice, or sugar in your coffee in the morning. All will boost your energy for a short time, but the sugar rebound they cause will make you crave sugar the rest of the day.

2. Recharge your battery at night if your desire is to have all-day energy. Go to bed earlier—even a half-hour can help.

3. Avoid exposure to electronic screens (TV, computer or video games) before bed. Bright light to the eyes can simulate daylight and keep you awake longer. Changes in light exposure (too much light at night when your body expects darkness, something shift workers experience) appear to have a biological or hormonal effect that is still not fully understood.

4. Train your body to drink more water. By the time you're thirsty you are already dehydrated, and that puts you at risk for daytime fatigue and a lack of focus and concentration. It may take you a few weeks to get used to drinking more water, so take about three weeks to work up to eight 8-ounce glasses per day.

Sam actually felt better the day after he started his new program. Once you start giving your body what it needs, it responds quickly.

# Tired? You might be thirsty.

## WHAT:

You're eating high-energy foods and sleeping well. So why are you so tired? You might be thirsty. Our bodies are more than 70 percent water, yet most people drink very little water each day. In fact, most office workers drink only coffee, tea and soda during a typical workday.

## WHY:

Dehydration is one of the primary causes of day-time fatigue. All body functions require water, and if you are not drinking enough of it, your body and mind will not work as they should, affecting everything from blood pressure to muscle contractions. Even a small deficiency of body water can trigger fuzzy short-term memory and difficulty focusing on a computer screen or printed words. One-third of Americans mistake thirst for hunger because their thirst mechanism is so weak or misunderstood.

Transform Your Health
in 60 Seconds a Day

# HOW:

- Drink a glass of water as soon as you get up. After a month of doing this, you will have trained your body to be thirsty upon waking.

- Keep a bottle of water everywhere—car, desk, briefcase—even in the bathroom, since you'll be spending a lot of time in there.

- If you don't like the taste of water, add a squirt of lemon or lime.

- Cut back on caffeine. It takes 2 cups of water to replace the fluid lost from every cup of a caffeinated drink.

- Hang in there. I know you will feel as if you are living in your bathroom; it will take about two to three weeks to train your body to urinate less often.

# Lunch-time rocket fuel

## WHAT:

You slept late and skipped breakfast. Now it's time for lunch and you are ravenous. What can you eat that will boost your energy and won't slow you down for the rest of the day?

## WHY:

Overeating at lunch, and eating the wrong foods, will set up your body for the perfect afternoon nap. If a nap isn't an option for you, you will need to learn to add high-energy foods to your lunch to boost your afternoon energy and your brainpower.

Transform Your Health
in 60 Seconds a Day

# HOW:

 Avoid high-sugar foods and excess fat.

 Make veggies a big part of your meal.

 Cut back on carbs and include more veggies and protein.

How to apply the above recommendations to popular lunches:

**Sandwich.** Remove some of the meat and cheese; eat the sandwich open-faced if feeling really tired (carbs can relax you and make you tired). Add some fiber, such as a whole apple or veggie salad, to help keep your energy steady.

**Chinese food.** Skip the fried rice and chow mein. Eat as many veggies as you want. Protein and rice should each take up about 25 percent of the space on your plate. Brown rice will boost your energy more than white.

**Mexican food.** Fajitas are a good choice. Eat all the veggies; your protein should take up about 25 percent of your plate. Black or pinto beans are better for your energy than refried (too much fat). Choose either a tortilla or rice, but not both (too many carbs). Sour cream and cheese (too much fat) are also energy zappers.

Always have on hand a high-fiber, high-energy snack that can help increase the energy you get from your lunch. Some examples are: piece of fruit, carrot sticks, edamame (fresh soybeans).

# Snacking is as important as a great night's sleep.

### WHAT:

You wake up energized but by mid-morning you're feeling hungry, grumpy and tired. And since our bodies were designed to get tired about eight hours after waking—nature's way of making sure we rest and take care of ourselves—you hit another slump in the afternoon. For those times when rest isn't an option, having a high-energy snack can get you over your energy crisis and back to productivity.

### WHY:

It's simple—when your blood sugar drops, your energy drops. Low blood sugar makes it almost impossible to be focused and productive. If your blood sugar stays low for too long, recovering your energy may be difficult, even if you do eat a good snack.

Transform Your Health
in 60 Seconds a Day

# HOW:

 Eat some protein. Protein creates a substance in your body called catecholamines, which make you feel a bit more assertive and energetic.

 Here are a few of my favorite high-protein snacks: one palmful of trail mix; a small packet of string cheese; a tablespoon of peanut butter; a slice of lunch meat; a hard-boiled egg (components of the egg can also be very calming for your brain, great if you have a stressful afternoon ahead); smoked salmon on a cracker; a small piece of turkey jerky; edamame; a cup of hot chicken broth; a small can of tuna or half of a high-protein energy bar (avoid the ones with maltitol; it's a laxative!).

 Eat more protein and less sugar at breakfast. Animal protein at breakfast will keep your energy up all day. Then focus on small snacks throughout the day to keep your energy high. (See chapters "The only food plan you'll ever need" on page 28 and "What to do when fast food is the only food" on page 94 for healthy snack ideas and why snacking is so important for sustained energy.)

 Cut out any sugary drinks during your day and replace them with water or green tea—iced or hot. Green tea has a form of caffeine that kicks in in the afternoon and helps keep your energy up. (See the chapter "Green tea gets the green light" on page 126 for more information about the benefits of green tea.)

 Eat your small high-protein snack outside. Spending even a few minutes outside can really increase your energy and focus.

# Make your bed or make your breakfast?

## WHAT:

It's another crazy morning, and you have a choice: make your bed or make your breakfast. On the one hand, it's nice to come home to a tidy house. But if you don't eat breakfast you could gain weight today and your math skills may not be as sharp.

## WHY:

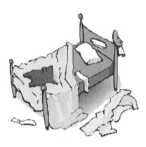

Breakfast skippers are more likely to have more body fat than their breakfast-eating counterparts. They will be more likely to gorge (not just overeat, but gorge) later in the day and will burn approximately 150 fewer calories each day. Do the math: One hundred fifty calories multiplied by 365 days a year is a body-fat gain of more than 15 pounds a year. In addition to carrying more body fat, breakfast skippers will also be more likely to experience poor and delayed decision-making skills.

Transform Your Health
in 60 Seconds a Day

# HOW:

 Your best breakfast needs to have three components: protein (at least 5–7 grams), fiber (at least 3 grams) and some fat. All three will keep you full, and the protein will help your brain focus. If you eat a fat-free breakfast, you are likely to be hungry within two hours.

 Here are some of my favorite protein-fiber-fat-combo breakfast ideas:

1. Whole grain toast, peanut butter and an apple

2. Banana and half a protein bar

3. Eggs with whole-grain toast and fruit

4. Oatmeal with a handful of berries and some nuts

5. Cold cereal (low sugar and high fiber) with some fruit and low-fat (not nonfat) milk or soymilk

 Train yourself to be hungry in the morning. Most people aren't hungry then because they've eaten too much the night before. Cut back on your dinner, and within a few weeks your morning hunger will return.

# Popeye always had energy!

## WHAT:

You're feeling run-down and weak. You are also looking a bit pale and pasty. If you're eating a balanced diet and sleeping well, your fatigue could be due to an iron deficiency.

## WHY:

Iron helps ensure that you have enough energy to make it through your day. It also plays a role in keeping your immune system in top form and your brain functioning at top speed. Iron's main function is to carry oxygen to cells in the body. Not enough oxygen? Then you will feel run-down and fatigued. And if you starve your cells of oxygen for too long, cell damage could occur.

Your body absorbs iron from foods, but this is not an easy task. You can increase iron absorption *sixfold* by adding some vitamin C to your meals that contain iron.

Transform Your Health
in 60 Seconds a Day

# HOW:

 Add a handful of berries to iron-fortified cereal.

 Eat an apple or orange after lunch or dinner.

 Have some strawberries on top of your spinach salad.

 Eat a peach with a handful of trail mix.

 Add a squirt of lemon to your iced tea drunk with a meal.

 For women only: add a daily multivitamin with iron to your after-breakfast routine.

 For men only: Men don't need to help their bodies absorb iron, since iron deficiency isn't a problem for them. Having the opposite situation of women, men need to be cautious about consuming too much iron and should avoid multivitamins that contain it.

# Sleep, can you ever get enough?

## WHAT:

Sleep, or lack thereof, is something that more than 50 percent of Americans have trouble with at least a few times each week. When you frequently get less sleep than your body needs, you are setting yourself up for a slower metabolism (you can gain weight if you sleep less than six and a half hours per night), an accelerated aging process and, possibly, the early stages of diabetes. Chronic sleep debt can also speed up age-related health problems such as high blood pressure, obesity and even memory loss.

**Can you catch up on the weekends?**

You can make up some sleep-debt damage by spending longer than eight hours in bed when time allows. Sneak in sleep where you can; napping is helpful!

## WHY:

In the last 100 years, the average night's sleep has diminished from over nine hours to less than seven and a half hours. While we each have different requirements, you should shoot for a minimum of seven and a half hours, but eight or nine is even better. During a good night's sleep, your body has a chance to strengthen your immune system, repair your muscle tissue, deposit calcium into your bones, activate your long-term memory, replenish your brain chemicals, grow your hair and renew your skin cells.

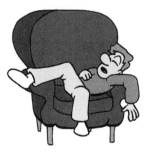

Transform Your Health
in 60 Seconds a Day

# HOW...

## ... to fall asleep faster and stay asleep:

 Wear socks to bed. When you lie down your body prepares for sleep by distributing heat from your core out to the fingers and toes. By warming up your feet, you signal your body that it's time for sleep.

 Wear an eye mask. Sleeping in complete darkness signals your body to produce more melatonin, the hormone that helps you sleep, so you can fall asleep faster and sleep more deeply. It doesn't take much light to "turn off" this process, so get rid of your night light and don't turn on any lights if you need to take a potty break.

 No electronic screens of any kind! That's right; avoid computer, TV and video-game screens before bed. The light from these screens signals your body that it is still daytime, and this may keep you from producing melatonin.

 Avoid alcohol. Yes, I know it does relax you enough to fall asleep, but have you ever noticed that a few hours later you wake up? After you metabolize the alcohol, your blood sugar drops and you wake up with a start!

# Can't sleep?
# Go munch on some cherries!

## WHAT:

It's cherry season. I've been eating some every day, and I've been sleeping great. I just read some research about cherries and their link with a restful night of sleep (Hattori and others 1995). They contain a substance that can regulate your sleep cycle and enable you to sleep better. It turns out there are many foods that can help you get a great night's sleep.

## WHY:

Many of us rely on over-the-counter or prescription medication to help us sleep. Many of these may cause next day grogginess or dehydration. Why not try an alternative that is healthy and has with no side effects?

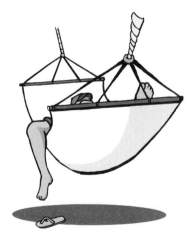

Transform Your Health
in 60 Seconds a Day

# HOW:

**Cherries** not only contain melatonin, a substance that helps regulate your sleep cycle, they also contain an ibuprofen-like substance that works as an anti-inflammatory, or analgesic. This substance helps reduce arthritis pain. It also lowers uric acid levels, which lessens the pain of gout.

(Besides helping promote sleep, cherries also have many anti-cancer properties, and a substance in cherry juice can help prevent tooth decay!)

**Sleep Teas** help you fall asleep naturally. One of them, chamomile, contains a substance known to induce calm and promote sleep. A word of caution, though: Chamomile is in the ragweed family, and ragweed is a common allergen. After drinking many cups of this tea before bed, I would get sleepy and then be so stuffy I couldn't breathe! There are other "sleepy teas" on the market that don't contain chamomile, so check labels.

**Passionflower** is an herb that was used by the Aztecs as a sedative. It is a sleep inducer and creates a sense of relaxation and euphoria. Passionflower was also used during World War II by the Germans as a "truth serum." You can find passionflower in both tea and tincture form. Follow the instructions on the label.

# Section 3:
# The Wonderful World of Fruits and Veggies

# Section 3: The Wonderful World of Fruits and Veggies

I grew up on a small ranch, and mine was the typical meat-and-potatoes family. Fruits and veggies were not featured at our meals. Though my mom always packed a piece of fruit in my school lunches, in 12 years I never ate any of it. I finally ate my first apple in college, my first apple not enclosed in pie crust! A friend handed it to me during a road trip, and I remember being perplexed and thinking: "We have potato chips too; why would I forego the chips for this thing?" I ate the apple so my friends wouldn't think I was strange; after all, I was a getting my degree in Health Science.

Ten years ago, when I finally got serious about my health, I knew it was time to get serious about adding more healthful foods to my diet. I was doing all right with veggies, but I just wasn't eating fruit. At first I had to force myself to eat one piece of it a day, but then one became two, and next thing I knew I was actually craving the stuff.

Eating fruits and veggies is nature's way of keeping us healthy. They contain vitamin C, potassium and lycopene—to name just a few of their nutrients—which act as our personal wellness-security systems. Most Americans consume fewer than two fruit and veggie servings a day, not nearly enough to ward off common illnesses, much less strengthen our immune systems for long-term wellness and disease prevention.

Transform Your Health
in 60 Seconds a Day

This section will help you understand further why fruits and veggies are so important for maintaining health, and you'll learn how to sneak more of them into your daily diet. For starters, always keep one fruit snack sitting on your desk (as a good reminder) and the other in a drawer (so nobody takes it).

Believe me, if I succeeded in turning fruits and veggies into treats, so can you!

# Fruits and veggies versus cancer

## WHAT:

Cancer doesn't develop overnight. It typically takes two to three decades, or in some cases four or five, for a healthy cell to morph into a cancerous tumor. This means you have many years to starve or feed it.

> "The more fruits and vegetables people eat, the less likely they are to get cancer, from colon and stomach to breast and even lung cancer. For many cancers, *persons with high fruit and vegetable intake have about half the risk of people with low intakes.*"
>
> (Greenwald 2002)

## WHY:

Antioxidants and vitamins in our food can kick out carcinogens, repair cellular damage and even shrink pre-cancerous cells. As little as one serving of a fruit or veggie a day can be protective against cancer, but the more of them you eat, the greater the protection benefit. One recent study (Schabath and Spitz, 2006) found that two fruits or veggies a day could increase your protection from lung cancer by 46 percent!

The latest recommendations suggest that two to three servings of fruits or veggies each day are very disease-protective.

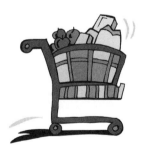

# HOW:

Science is constantly changing, and every day a discovery is made that sends nutritionists in all directions. For example, a few years ago very few nutritionists would have encouraged their clients to eat melons, especially watermelon, due to their low nutrient content. Current research really blows that theory out of the water! We now know that watermelons have more lycopene, a prostate-cancer preventer, than tomatoes, previously believed to be the best source.

While the research may vary slightly, the majority of it agrees that fruits and veggies with a high level of vitamin C are among the best cancer fighters. Your best bet is to pick at least two servings a day.

Here are some of your best choices to increase your vitamin C:

- Cantaloupe
- Papaya
- Strawberries
- Kiwi
- Orange
- Grapefruit
- Other citrus fruits, including squeezing lemon in your water
- Orange and yellow bell peppers
- Broccoli
- Collard or mustard greens
- Spinach
- Tomatoes
- Parsley

# The Krazy Glue-vitamin C connection

In the previous chapter, I told you that vitamin C protects against cancer. Read on for more ways this vitamin helps keep you healthy.

## WHAT:

It's true, vitamin C is similar to Krazy Glue. It holds your body together. Not only that, **"Getting 300 mg of vitamin C daily can add six years to a man's life and two years to a woman's life."** (Enstrom 1992)

## WHY:

Vitamin C keeps your cells healthy and thriving. And, since there are cells throughout your entire body, it is crucial that you have plenty of "glue" in those cells to keep your body healthy, functioning and upright!

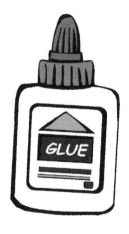

The government recommends we get 60 milligrams a day. Most nutrition researchers agree that is too little. Dr. Linus Pauling, a pioneer of vitamin-C research, advocated upwards of thousands of milligrams daily just for basic health and much more if you were sick with a cold or the flu or had a chronic disease. Vitamin C is an extremely powerful antioxidant and our first line of defense against free radicals. Free radicals are what make us age; they might be pollution, alcohol, drugs or smoking. They circulate in our body, waging war on our healthy cells. Vitamin C traps and annihilates these bad guys.

Here are a few other reasons not to skip the "C":

1. It helps protect your joints from rheumatoid arthritis. According to a recent study, "A diet low in fruits and veggies doubled the likelihood of arthritis; low C nearly quadrupled the risk." (Pattison and others 2004)

2. It protects your gums from disease, receding and bleeding.

3. It helps reduce swelling and supports the growth of connective tissue.

# HOW:

Your body needs different levels of vitamin C throughout the day. If your day is particularly stressful, your body's need for C will greatly increase. Here are a few other daily "stressors" that will increase your body's requirement for vitamin C:

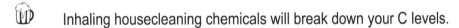 Inhaling housecleaning chemicals will break down your C levels.

Drinking alcohol (even one drink) will lower C levels.

Smoking will really annihilate your C!

The most surprising hit to your vitamin C levels? Walking in and out of an air-conditioned room or car.

Some of the best sources of vitamin C are fruits and veggies. To keep your cell "glue" functioning as it should, include at least two of them daily. See the previous chapter, "Fruits and veggies versus cancer," for some good choices.

# An apple a day

## WHAT:

It's not glamorous like a pineapple or exciting like a fresh, juicy peach, but the apple is still one of my favorite fruits. For one thing, it's consistent. It doesn't matter what the season, you can still get a great-tasting apple.

## WHY:

According to the National Institutes of Health, the less fiber you get in your diet, the more likely you are to gain weight. The recommended amount of fiber we should eat each day is 25–30 grams. Most Americans average around 15 grams.

One of the other reasons that I eat at least one apple a day is because it helps protect my lungs. I had asthma as a kid, and apples have been shown to be very beneficial for people who have lung disease.

Here are a few other reasons that I love the humble little apple!

- Apple polyphenols, substances that contribute to your good health, can help lower cholesterol, increase antioxidant capacity and decrease your risk of chronic diseases such as cardiovascular disease, cancer, asthma and diabetes.

- Apples contain a variety of phytochemicals, including quercetin, catechin, and phloridzin, all of which are strong antioxidants. (For more about phytochemicals, see the chapter "Meet the phytochemicals. No, they're not the latest rock band!" on page 114.)

- Apples have excellent free-radical-scavenging properties. When an old car sits out in the rain, free radi-

Transform Your Health in 60 Seconds a Day

cals make it get rusty. Apples help keep you from getting "rusty" on the inside!

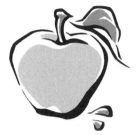

- Thanks in part to their high soluble fiber content, apples will keep you fuller longer. Soluble fiber absorbs water and delays the emptying of the stomach. These fibers also keep you from absorbing all the fat from meals!

# HOW:

Apples can stay in your car or desk for a week and still taste pretty good. Get in the habit of eating one at lunch every day or on the way home from work.

# The power of fruit, not fruit juice

## WHAT:

Many nutritionists will say that fruit juice is an excellent way to help hit your goal of five fruits and veggies each day. Nutritionally, fruit and veggie juices have some similarities to the real thing, but when you really compare the whole food to the juice, the juice doesn't stack up.

## WHY:

A study in the journal Pediatrics (Welsh and others 2005), found that preschool children who drank more than 12 ounces of juice a day were three times more likely to be overweight than kids who didn't drink juice (12 ounces is equivalent to one and a half cups, or approximately two boxes, of juice).

A piece of fruit has an incredible abundance of cancer fighters in its skin and flesh, and it's impossible to transfer all of these into a glass.

Juice can also make your blood sugar rise dramatically since it has no fiber to slow down its absorption into your bloodstream. In fact, diabetics should avoid most fruit juices for this reason. (If a juice contains pulp, as in some orange juice, the blood-sugar rise is less dramatic.) Since very few Americans come close to eating the recommended 25–30 grams of fiber a day, a piece of fruit can go a long way in helping to meet that number.

Making juice from whole fruit concentrates the fruit sugars and really increases the calorie content. Some food manufacturers also add a lot of sugars to juice to change the taste. Also, many "juice" drinks have less than 10 percent real juice—so much for getting a good dose of vitamins from your juice.

Transform Your Health
in 60 Seconds a Day

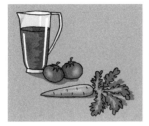 Don't get me wrong; juice can serve an important role in your nutrition program. It's an acceptable substitute if you don't have a lot of fresh fruit around or if you're traveling and can't find fruit in a restaurant.

## HOW:

While juice can be a good addition to your nutritional menu occasionally, pick the fruit at least twice a day!

# If a bug wouldn't eat it, then neither should you!

According to a study by The Environmental Working Group (www.ewg.org 2006):

"People can lower their pesticide exposure by 90 percent by avoiding the top 12 most contaminated fruits and vegetables and eating the least contaminated instead. Eating the 12 most contaminated fruits and vegetables will expose a person to nearly 20 pesticides per day, on average. Eating the 12 least contaminated will expose a person to a fraction over 2 pesticides per day."

## WHAT:

Pesticides are designed to kill. They are toxic to bugs, weeds and anything else that might eat food intended for you, and they can be toxic to you too. The risks of consuming pesticides depend on many factors, including the toxicity of the pesticide, amount of exposure, your age and lifetime exposure to other toxins.

## WHY:

A small dose of pesticide can harm people, especially during childhood and critical periods of fetal development, and the effects may be long-lasting. Because long-term effects are not known, it's best to minimize your exposure. Even small changes in eating habits can greatly diminish your exposure to these toxins.

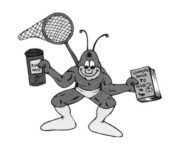

Transform Your Health in 60 Seconds a Day

# HOW:

**Avoid the 12 most contaminated fruits and veggies:**

Apples, bell peppers, celery, cherries, grapes (imported), nectarines, peaches, pears potatoes, spinach, strawberries and raspberries

In the study cited on the previous page, peaches and raspberries were found to have the most pesticides, with nine on a single sample, followed by strawberries and apples, with eight.

These fruits and veggies are very important to include in your diet, and this study is not trying to discourage you from consuming them. But it does clearly state that if you can, buy organic to reduce the risk of extra toxins building up in your body. If organically grown produce is difficult to find, try farmers markets and health food stores. You can also purchase frozen organic berries for those dark days of winter when you're getting fed up with eating just apples and bananas.

**The 12 least contaminated fruits and veggies:**

Asparagus, avocados, bananas, broccoli, cauliflower, sweet corn, kiwi, mangos, onions, papaya, pineapples and peas

According to the study, these 12 fruits and veggies are safe to consume even if not grown organically.

Please note that in this study the researchers did wash the produce. What they discovered is that while washing helps reduce some pesticide exposure, it in no way eliminates the majority of it, since much of the pesticide is retained within the cells of the produce.

# Hungry? Go eat some sunscreen!

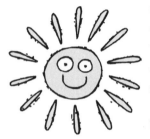

## WHAT:

Skin cancer rates have doubled in the U.S. since 1973, so protecting your skin from the sun is a health issue we should all be concerned about. In a study reported in the American Journal of Clinical Nutrition (Stahl and others 2000), people who took a beta carotene supplement suffered less reddening of the skin and less skin damage than those subjects who did not take the supplement.

## WHY:

The American Institute for Cancer Research suggests that a diet high in fruits and veggies can be somewhat skin-protective and may be a nice "addition" to the sunscreen you are already using. (If you're not using one, buy one today!) (Zsuzsanna and others 2003). According to the researchers in the American Journal of Clinical Nutrition study above, eating more beta carotene-rich fruits and veggies may increase your skin's own natural protection by 2 or 3 SPF (sun protection factor, the rating system for sunscreen). While this increase is not going to keep your skin from burning, when combined with sunscreen, it will really boost your skin protection.

Transform Your Health
in 60 Seconds a Day

# HOW:

Increase your consumption of beta carotene-rich foods: peaches, cherries, papaya, carrots and any other orange or yellow fruits and veggies.

 Add frozen pineapple or mango to a smoothie.

 Drink a peach margarita or daiquiri (while high in calories, it still counts!)

 Take a bag of carrot sticks or sliced orange or yellow bell peppers to work.

 Add pureed pumpkin to bread or muffin mix.

# French fries are not veggies!

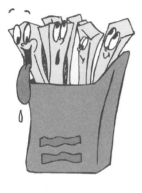

### WHAT:

Today, one out of nine American adults will not include one fruit or veggie in their diet, and only 50 percent of American children will eat one serving of a fruit or veggie.

### WHY:

The vitamins from fruits and veggies are some of the most powerful disease fighters available. According to the American Cancer Society, almost one-third of all cancers could be prevented by eating a healthy diet. When most of us think about adding more veggies or fruits into our diets we think salads—**BORING!** There are so many ways to add more fruits and veggies into your diet; it just takes a little creativity!

## HOW:

Here are some simple and creative ways to increase your fruit and veggie intake:

 Add some grated carrot or zucchini to your favorite muffin recipe.

 Add corn kernels or chopped peppers to cornbread mix.

 Puree a bag of frozen broccoli or peas and add to soups and pasta sauce.

 Add grated carrots to twice-baked potatoes (it looks just like cheese!).

Transform Your Health
in 60 Seconds a Day

Add leftover veggies to canned soups.

Top pancakes, French toast or oatmeal with berries.

Add berries to ice cream or frozen yogurt.

Add coleslaw to green or pasta salads.

Get a small fruit smoothie in the morning and drink it throughout the day.

Try low-sodium tomato juice as a mid-morning snack.

Keep carrot sticks or snap peas and low-cal dressing at your office and home.

Add pre-chopped onions and garlic to stir-fries, salads and pasta sauce.

Roast veggies (about 45 minutes at 375º) and add to sandwiches, sauces and salads.

Herbs are also healthy additions to your diet, as they contain disease-fighting phytochemicals (see the chapter "Spice up your life" on page 74), so think about adding cilantro or parsley to salads, and rosemary to roasted potatoes.

# Holiday fruitcake or medical miracle?

## WHAT:

Fruitcake may not improve your holiday health, but fresh fruit might. During the holiday season we are exposed to more cold and flu viruses, more alcohol, sugar and fat than at other times of the year. For those of us, including me, who don't like to turn down the extra serving of pumpkin pie, here are a few holiday fruit remedies that may help you avoid some common holiday ailments.

## WHY:

During the holidays many of us skip the foods that may make us feel better and keep us healthy. There are so many other items to choose from that the lowly fruit gets pushed aside for more interesting and traditional holiday goodies.

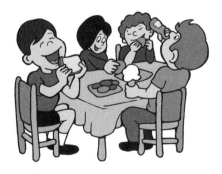

# HOW...
## ... can fruit help you feel better?

 **Bloating!** Who hasn't felt that horrible morning-after bloat? Your eyes are puffy and you can't zip up your pants. **The Remedy:** Eat more citrus fruit. Oranges, grapefruits and lemons can help draw the extra fluid out of your body. This works best in the evening before you go to bed. Eat an orange or drink some water with lemon, and you'll wake up feeling better. This really can be an overnight remedy to excess water weight!

 **Upset tummy?** Your stomach is bloated and you have uncomfortable gas (well, I guess it's never comfortable). **The Remedy:** Eat some pineapple. Pineapple contains bromelain, which acts as a stomach enzyme and helps digest food. As we age, our digestion becomes less efficient at breaking down food. When we overeat, the stomach gets overwhelmed and needs some reinforcements. Try a slice or two of pineapple after your holiday (or anytime) meal.

 **Have you gained a few holiday pounds?** The average American gains 5 pounds between Halloween and the Super Bowl. Don't let this happen to you! **The Remedy:** Eat an apple before lunch and dinner, and you may lose up to two pounds a week. Increasing your fiber intake before a meal will create a feeling of fullness, curbing your appetite before you hit the holiday buffet.

 **I'm in a bad mood!** Who hasn't had a few cranky moments over the holidays? Most of us just push through it and keep on going. But there is a fruit solution to holiday (or anytime) grumpiness and depression—citrus fruits. Smelling a lemon, or any citrus fruit, may help lift depression or shift moods. **The Remedy:** Add the juice of half a lemon to a glass of water or a cup of hot herbal tea. You'll inhale the citrus scent as you drink. It's worth a try!

# Section 4:
# Health Tip Potluck

# Section 4: Health Tip Potluck

Bob felt that if he ate one more airline meal he was going to crack. He traveled at least once a week, often through two or three time zones and back in days. He followed a great health routine at home, but traveling was another story. He was often in a rush to get to the airport, so he would throw something to snack on (usually a meal replacement bar) into his briefcase and run out the door. With fewer airlines serving meals these days, his only food for hours would be that small snack from home and as many packets of peanuts or pretzels he could get from the flight attendants.

Bob successfully implemented many of the health habits in this section while on the go.

This is the section for those who feel they eat pretty well but still don't enjoy the health they want. This "potluck" of health information and issues—from why eggs really are good for you to why airplane water really isn't—will help you make the healthiest choices when you are faced with situations that may challenge your best intentions to take good care of yourself. Sometimes we just need to tweak our routines a little to improve our health a lot.

# They're small, tasty and cheap!

## WHAT:

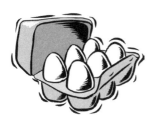

Eggs! I know what you're thinking: "Eggs are bad for you!" And up until a few years ago, nutritionists told the public to limit its intake. But the good news is that the humble egg has been let out of nutrition purgatory, and for some very good reasons.

In the 1970s, the media reported that eating eggs raises cholesterol. This information was based on research that looked at the effect of *dried* egg yolks on cholesterol levels. The misconstrued message took, and many of us started shunning eggs. But it turns out that, while eating dried egg yolks may raise cholesterol, real eggs don't. Thirty years of research has shown that eating dietary cholesterol from eggs has only a small effect on raising our cholesterol levels. Eggs contain very little saturated fat, which makes their impact on blood cholesterol different from foods such as red meat or buttery pastries.

# WHY...
## ... you want to eat them:

Eggs are:

- Packed with protein, minerals, and vitamins, A, D, E and B

- Low in calories, only about 75 per serving

- Rich in essential minerals

- Packed with lutein—the nutrient responsible for preventing age-related macular degeneration

- Full of trace elements, including iron and zinc, which help form red blood cells and boost immunity

Eggs also have a brain-calming effect, due to the lecithin they contain, and are a great choice in the morning if you have a stressful day ahead of you.

# HOW:

Purchase free-range, omega-3-fortified eggs. Free-range eggs, compared to conventionally produced ones, have higher levels of omega-3 fatty acids, and free-range hens are treated in a humane manner—another good reason to buy free-range. Omega-3 polyunsaturated fatty acids play an integral role in cell-membrane function and development of the brain and eyes. Additional benefits include reduced risk of heart disease and, possibly, a reduced likelihood of behavioral problems, depression and inflammatory conditions such as rheumatoid arthritis. Here are some easy ways to add eggs to your diet:

- A hard-boiled egg as a mid-morning or -afternoon snack will give you sustained and boundless energy for a few hours.

- An egg on toast is a great breakfast choice. In fact, recent research has shown that dieters who start their day with an egg lose more weight faster—and keep it off (Vander Wal and others 2005).

- A hard-boiled egg in your lunch salad will give you a high-protein, energy-producing lunch.

# Spice up your life

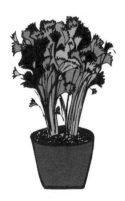

## WHAT:

When most of us think about herbs or spices we think about taste, not health. But spices and herbs have been shown to have medicinal qualities, along with providing a huge antioxidant hit. In some cases, herbs have more antioxidants than the foods they are added to.

## WHY:

Spices and herbs, with no side effects and minimal cost, can provide remedies for many health problems, such as nausea, diarrhea, anxiety, congestion and diabetes.

## HOW...
## ...to incorporate herbs and spices into your eating plan:

**Rosemary** is perfect for use with roasted potatoes and other veggies. Also use it in your marinade for grilled meats. When grilled, beef, poultry and pork create carcinogenic compounds called heterocyclic amines. When researchers added a bit of rosemary to the meat while grilling, fewer carcinogens were formed (Nerurkar and others 2005). So, while this herb can make your food taste better, it will also keep it safer.

**Parsley** is great for digestion and getting rid of excess water weight. Add chopped Italian flat-leaf parsley to salads or soups, or even put it in a sandwich. Parsley is also a great breath freshener at the end of a meal.

**Ginger** works well for nausea and upset stomach. It's also an anti-inflammatory, which means it may be useful in fighting heart disease, cancer,

Alzheimer's disease and arthritis. Plus, it's high in antioxidants that fight all kinds of diseases. You can brew some ginger tea (available in supermarkets), or suck on some ginger hard candy. You can also grate up fresh ginger to use in marinades for meat, fish and vegetables. **Interesting tidbit**: The health benefits of ginger were documented over 2,000 years ago!

**Cinnamon.** A study in the Journal of Nutrition found that of all spices, cinnamon is one of the richest sources of disease-fighting antioxidants (Mancini and others 1998). It has been used as an anti-microbial to stop the growth of bacteria, fungi and yeast. It has been used as an anti-inflammatory. It also has anti-clotting properties, which help prevent unwanted clumping of blood platelets. And, it may help boost brain function.

One of the most amazing findings for cinnamon has been its effect on lowering blood sugar levels. A study published in the journal Diabetes Care found that half a teaspoon of cinnamon a day significantly reduced blood sugar levels in those with type 2 diabetes (Khan and others 2003). It also reduced triglyceride levels, LDL (bad) cholesterol and total cholesterol levels.

Sprinkle a little cinnamon on fresh fruit and yogurt, or break up a cinnamon stick and place it in your coffee maker with the grounds. Not only will your coffee taste great and have some added health effects, it will make the whole house smell wonderful.

**Oregano:** Two of oregano's compounds, thymol and carvacrol, have potent antibacterial properties. Oregano is also a potent antioxidant, rich in phytonutrients (plant nutrients).

On a per-gram basis, the antioxidant activity of fresh oregano is:

- 42 times greater than that of apples
- 30 times greater than that of potatoes
- 12 times greater than that of oranges
- 4 times greater than that of blueberries

Add fresh or dried oregano to Italian dishes, salad dressings, egg dishes, vegetables, meats and more.

# Oh, nuts!

## WHAT:

For years, I told my weight-loss clients: "Whatever you do, don't eat nuts." Nuts used to be something to be avoided. But I'm here to eat some crow, along with a handful of almonds, to tell you that eating nuts (after all, people have been doing it for thousands of years) is good for your health and can help you lose weight.

## WHY:

Many nutritionists consider nuts to have more nutritional value than meats or grains. They are full of antioxidants (consider each nut to be a tiny antioxidant pill), vitamins and minerals. They also have a dose of heart-healthy fat and some protein. Here are some health benefits of some common nuts:

**ALMONDS:** Eating a small handful of these nuts each day has been shown to dramatically reduce cholesterol levels. Snacking on almonds on a daily basis may protect you against heart disease and diabetes.

**PEANUTS:** Although not technically a nut, peanuts (and peanut butter), eaten daily, can help lower LDL cholesterol and triglycerides. (See the chapter "Eat to fill and thrill!" on page 6 for the connection between eating peanuts and losing weight.)

Also, because of their high fat content, nuts go rancid quickly, so store them (unshelled, if possible) in the refrigerator until you're ready to eat them. Just about any type of nut is fine—just eat them as unprocessed as possible. Raw is best.

Transform Your Health
in 60 Seconds a Day

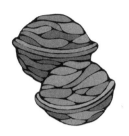

**WALNUTS:** These nuts have been shown to protect your cardiovascular system, even if you abuse it with a high-fat diet. These little nuts appear to take care of your body, even when you're not.

**PISTACHIOS:** An ounce of pistachios has more fiber than a half-cup of spinach! These nuts are a great addition to your diet on those days when you haven't eaten enough fiber.

# HOW:

Eating nuts is probably the easiest suggestion in this book to follow. I wish I could tell you to eat bags of them each day, but a serving size—about an ounce—fits in the palm of your hand, like an airplane bag of peanuts. I like to have my clients measure out a shot-glass worth of nuts into a small snack bag to help keep portions under control.

# Beans: great for health, bad for relationships?

## WHAT:

Beans are one of nature's almost-perfect foods, full of vitamins, protein and—no surprise—fiber. Most nutritionists consider beans to be the healthiest and most economical protein on the planet. Americans used to eat more of them, but as we have gotten more prosperous beans have been replaced with animal protein.

## WHY:

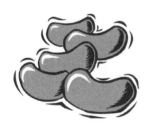

Beans lower cholesterol, fight heart disease and diabetes, decrease hypertension and stabilize blood sugar. In one study, participants who ate beans four times a week had a 22 percent lower risk of heart disease (Bazzano and others 2001). Eating more beans can also help preserve your bones. Animal protein leaches calcium out of your bones, while beans provide minerals that help your bones remain strong.

OK, let's tackle the delicate subject of what beans are really known for. It's true, beans are gas-producing. But the good news is that if you eat them often enough your body will learn to digest them and your "digestive challenge" will diminish. If the gas produced by beans remains a problem, try Beano, an enzyme product that can help reduce the gas.

Transform Your Health
in 60 Seconds a Day

# HOW...
## ...to add more beans to your diet:

Beans take a long time to cook, so if you're pressed for time, use canned beans. Because canned beans are usually full of sodium, though, throw them into a strainer and run cold water over them for 20 seconds and up to half the salt will be removed.

Eat more hummus. Hummus is a high-energy spread made from garbanzo beans. Use it on sandwiches, or dip veggies in it for a snack.

Top a salad with beans to help increase the protein content and, thus, your energy.

Complete the protein. Beans aren't a complete protein—they are missing two amino acids. These amino acids can easily be added by also eating a grain, nuts or a dairy product. For example, combining rice with beans completes the protein. You don't need to eat both items at the same meal, just on same day, to ensure you get the complete protein.

Eat beans three to four times each week. Half a cup is a serving.

# Hold the salt

## WHAT:

I love salty foods, but when I overindulge in them I make my body work harder. Our bodies are always trying to stay balanced, so if I eat too much salt, I will crave sweets until I am back in balance.

## WHY:

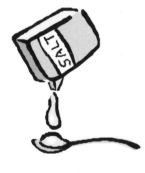

The majority of Americans are deficient in potassium, and one of the biggest problems with eating too much salt (sodium) is that it depletes your potassium levels. Depleted potassium levels can lead to these problems: cardiovascular disease, weak bones and fatigue. Americans' high consumption of processed foods is a major culprit, since most foods that come in a bag or a box are usually very high in sodium.

Do you have any idea what the biggest source of sodium is in the American diet? Bread! I'm not asking you to give up bread, but I am suggesting you begin to cut out some of the bagged and boxed foods that you eat on a daily basis.

Transform Your Health
in 60 Seconds a Day

# HOW:

To help prevent some of the above-mentioned diseases, along with feelings of constant fatigue (wouldn't it be great to have more energy naturally?), try to include some of the following foods:

**The Fruits**

Apricots, avocados, bananas, cantaloupe, dates, honeydew melon and citrus fruits

**The Veggies**

Asparagus, cauliflower, green beans, potatoes and winter squash

It's almost impossible to eat the necessary five to 10 servings of potassium-rich foods from just one food group, so it's best to choose a combination of fruits and veggies to hit your high potassium goal.

# The really big salad

## WHAT:

Remember that "Seinfeld" episode where Elaine searched high and low for "the really big salad"? The big salad is certainly the most popular lunch for women, but most women make the mistake of having it with a low- or no-fat dressing and little or no protein. Eating a lunch with little or no fat and protein will crank your sugar cravings into high gear.

## WHY:

Eating veggies at lunch is a good way to get vitamins, minerals and fiber. But if veggies are all you eat, your energy will last for less than an hour and you will find yourself needing sugar to regain your focus and concentration. You also need some fat with your salad to help your body absorb nutrients from the veggies.

According to the American Journal of Clinical Nutrition, people who consume salads with fat-free dressing absorb far fewer phytonutrients and vitamins than those who use a dressing containing fat (Brown and others 2004).

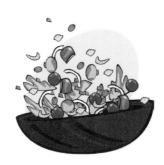

Transform Your Health
in 60 Seconds a Day

# HOW...

## ...to create a healthy and high-energy "big salad":

 Have a salad with at least five veggies (adding a fruit, such as a pear or apple, is great too).

 The darker the better! Though the most popular choice, salads made with iceberg lettuce take a nutritional back seat to salads made with dark or mixed greens. An iceberg-lettuce salad has 60-80 percent fewer nutrients than a salad made with raw spinach.

 Add a handful of chopped herbs to your salad to give it a flavor boost, along with a huge antioxidant hit. (See the chapter "Spice up your life" on page 74 for more about the health benefits of herbs.)

 Add some protein. It doesn't take much—a hard-boiled egg, a couple of slices of turkey breast or a half-cup of beans or lentils.

 Add some fat. Use healthy oil in your dressing, such as olive or grapeseed, to get the full nutritional benefit from your veggies. If you really do love the fat-free dressings, add fat to your salad by tossing in a palmful of nuts or seeds or a quarter of an avocado. That's enough to give your body the good fat and nutrition it craves.

# Hey, (taste) Bud!

## WHAT:

If you didn't have them, eating wouldn't be too exciting. Taste buds make life worth living! Perhaps that is an overstatement, but when you can't get some enjoyment out of eating, life doesn't seem as sweet. We each have about 10,000 taste buds on our tongues, and they are replaced every couple weeks. As we age, we lose about half of them, and I believe many of us compensate for this lack of taste sensation by trying to add in more flavor with excessive amounts of salt and sugar.

We have five types of taste buds: sweet, salty, bitter, sour and umani (savory).

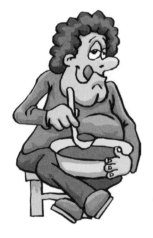

## WHY:

Each type of taste bud is located on a specific part of your tongue. Your sweet buds are located on the tip. So let's say you are eating a handful of really sweet grapes. If you eat them the traditional way, throwing them into your mouth toward the back of your throat, chances are your body will never really register that you are eating a sweet treat. What your body really wants you to do is smell the fruit first and then taste the sweetness on the tip of your tongue.

Transform Your Health
in 60 Seconds a Day

# HOW...
## ...to enjoy the food you eat more:

Take a good long whiff before eating your meal. Your sense of smell plays a huge role in how foods taste, so always try to pause and sniff your food—your taste buds will thank you for it!

Eat salty if you're craving something salty. Don't waste calories by trying other types of flavors.

Take smaller bites. They'll stimulate your taste buds more.

# Flying the not-so-friendly skies

## WHAT:

I have a stomachache, and I can almost pinpoint how I got it. I was on a plane and had just woken up from a nap, thirsty and dehydrated. The flight attendant poured me a cup of water from a pitcher. It tasted a bit off, but I just attributed that to my in-flight grogginess. It was only later (after half an hour of stomach cramps) that I realized the water poured for me was from a pitcher, not a bottle, and had come from the plane's water tank, which contained unfiltered and untested water.

## WHY...
## ...flying makes us tired and poses risks to our health:

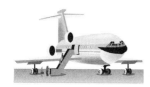

**The Water:** The water stored in airplane tanks can be full of bacteria and other undesirables. In fact, there are no government guidelines mandating water cleanliness or cleanliness of these tanks. Most pediatricians say never let your infant or child drink tap water on an airplane. Perhaps we adults shouldn't either.

**The Air:** Ever wonder why you fall asleep on take-off and then have a hard time getting back to sleep? Oxygen levels are lowest right before the plane takes off. When oxygen is low, you feel sleepy and groggy. If your goal is to sleep through your flight, set yourself up before take-off—use an eye mask and ear plugs, and buckle your seat belt

Transform Your Health
in 60 Seconds a Day

around your blanket so the attendant doesn't wake you to check it.

**Dehydration:** The humidity of most of the world's deserts is around 20 percent; optimal humidity for human comfort is about 50 percent. Airplane humidity can get as low as 5 percent on long flights. No wonder we get dehydrated, have dry skin and hair and even develop wrinkles while flying! It can take several days or more to recover your fluid balance, just in time for the flight home.

**Illness:** The poor quality of airplane air makes avoiding illness a real challenge. We get infected through the mucous membranes of the eyes, nose and mouth, and being dehydrated makes it easier for bugs to take hold.

**Inactivity:** Sitting still for hours at a time also poses risks to our health. When we don't move, our circulation is decreased, and this can lead to the formation of blood clots.

# HOW...

## ...to stay healthy in the air:

Keep the nose moist (I put moisturizer or lip balm around and slightly inside my nostrils).

Drink a glass of bottled water every hour while in the air, and keep it going after you land. It also helps to drink more water the day before the flight.

Bring a water atomizer and spray your face often to help keep your skin hydrated.

Don't drink the coffee or tea. They are made from the plane's water supply and don't get hot enough to kill harmful bacteria.

Don't drink alcohol! It will dehydrate you even more.

Accept bottled and canned drinks only.

Get up and move, or at least tap your toes and extend your legs forward, every hour to boost your circulation.

Never cross your legs—doing so cuts off circulation to the rest of your body.

Bring your own hand sanitizer to keep your hands clean.

Transform Your Health
in 60 Seconds a Day

# My "never" list

## WHAT:

I know, never say never. But I've gone and done it. You should never do or eat any of the following things. Research will back me up when I say that these things can really harm your health, in both the short and long term.

## WHY:

We are a society of convenience, but by making food preparation and access to food easier and faster, we have created ways to harm our bodies.

# HOW:

 **Never microwave in plastic.** When plastic is heated and comes into contact with food, especially fat, it releases toxins directly into the food. These toxins are then eaten and get stuck in your body. Most lodge in your fat cells, which means you carry them around for life. This plastic issue applies to all forms of plastic, from hard containers, to plastic plates, to plastic wrap.

**The fix:** Microwave food in glass containers and cover with paper towels or wax paper.

 **Never take vitamins on an empty stomach.** Vitamins need stomach acid to be digested properly. Without food in your stomach, you won't have enough stomach acid to break down the vitamins, and they will sit there, unabsorbed and possibly giving you an upset stomach, nausea and a headache.

**The fix:** Take your vitamins after meals. One of the easiest ways to do this is to keep some in your purse or briefcase and take them on your way back from lunch. To keep your vitamins potent, keep them out of the sun and heat.

 **Never eat THE GIANT PRETZEL.** At about 600 calories (just plain, no add-ons), this is a very high-calorie snack that will steal your energy almost as quickly as you eat it. It's a white-flour product, so it has about zero nutritional value, truly a filler food that just serves to "fill out" your jeans. This high-carb food creates massive amounts of serotonin (nature's Prozac) in your system, so a nap is about the only thing that sounds good after eating one. And because you just want to rest after eating one of these babies, guess where those calories get stored? Yup, right in your fat cells!

 Transform Your Health
in 60 Seconds a Day

**The fix:** Switch to a whole-grain pretzel, add loads of mustard for taste, and split it with a friend.

 **Never give in to THE MONSTER MALL COOKIE!** They taste great, and if they didn't cost about 800 calories apiece, I would spend more time shopping! These things are deadly; they will bring your energy up and then drop you down like a hot potato. The combo of the sugar and the carb will make you want to take a nap in the Nordstrom dressing room. Later in the day, you will find yourself craving salt (to balance out the sugar hit), and it will be hard to turn down that salty pretzel or hot dog (a vicious cycle).

**The fix:** Try the Mrs. Fields nibbler cookies; two weigh in at about 100 calories.

# Beat the heat

## WHAT:

People don't seem to take heat exhaustion seriously until it happens to them. Most of us have been there: It's August, you're outside working in the yard, and you're too dirty to go into the house for a glass of cold water. Next thing you know, you are nauseated, dizzy and have an intense headache. At this point most of us quit what we are doing and go inside to cool down. But those who keep at it are now at risk of heat stroke, which is extremely dangerous and possibly life-threatening.

## WHY:

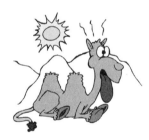

As our world gets warmer, we hear about more people, especially high-school athletes, dying from heat exposure. People of all ages are at risk of heat-related illness, whether working out strenuously or just puttering outside. The risk of heat illness goes up significantly if you have heart, lung or kidney disease or if you are overweight. Certain drugs can also increase your risk of heat illness, especially diuretics, tranquilizers, high blood pressure medicines and antidepressants. All of these inhibit your ability to sweat, which will send your internal temperature soaring. There are two different types of heat illness—heat exhaustion and heat stroke.

Symptoms of **heat exhaustion** are dizziness, weakness, nausea, headache, and cold and clammy skin.

Those with heat exhaustion should move to a cool area and rest with their head in a low position. They should drink plenty of cold water and put cold compresses to the back of their neck and to the forehead.

Symptoms of **heat stroke** are headache, numbness, confusion, elevated blood pressure and pulse rate, and profuse sweating.

Heat stroke is a medical emergency and requires rapid treatment to ensure the health of the victim. The sufferer must be immediately cooled in an ice bath to prevent further health implications.

# HOW...
## ...to reduce your risk of any heat-related illness:

 Drink plenty of water or other non-caffeinated beverages. Caffeinated beverages will dehydrate you and could increase your risk of heat illness.

 Get wet! While gardening in the heat, turn the hose on yourself. If out running, run through any sprinklers you see.

 Wear a breathable hat while exercising or gardening. Many hats today come with an SPF rating, so it's similar to wearing sunscreen. Find a hat that's not too tight and has vents to let in some air.

 Wear lightweight and loose clothing.

# What to do when fast food is the only food

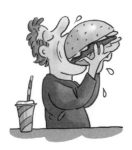

### WHAT:

It's lunchtime and you're stuck in your car. It appears that your only option is fast food. What do you choose?

### WHY:

Fast food is notorious for it's high fat, sodium, calories and large portions. It's the perfect lunch if you want to shut down your brain and take a long, restful nap and increase your risk of heart disease and high cholesterol. There is a way to make fast food work for you, though; you just don't want to make it a daily habit.

## HOW:

 Wendy's: chili and side salad.

 Mexican Restaurant: two bean burritos and piece of fruit.

 Pizza: First, load up on salad with at least five different kinds of veggies and some beans for more fiber. Order pizza with low-fat cheese, veggies and only one meat topping.

 Burger place: Get the smallest burger (no cheese), side salad and iced tea or water.

Transform Your Health
in 60 Seconds a Day

Sandwich shop: Order it on the thinnest bread they offer. Ask for double the veggies and less meat. Eat this with a small salad or tomato-based soup.

 Hot dog stand: Order the smallest dog they have, a chicken dog if possible. Eat this with a piece of fruit and a small bag of pretzels or baked chips.

 Juice smoothie: Order the smallest smoothie. Choose multiple fruits, no ice cream or sherbet, and an extra shot of protein and fiber.

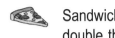 Coffee chain store: Low-fat or soymilk latté (they have less sugar than a mocha, and the milk has some protein), piece of fruit, small slice of low-fat nut or fruit bread.

Get in the habit of keeping high-fiber snacks with you to help bump up the nutrition and energy of fast foods. Fiber is the biggest factor missing from fast foods, so if you combine a high-fiber food with the above suggestions, you can make fast food a better high-energy lunch choice.

High fiber snack ideas:

 Trail mix with dried fruit and nuts

 Any fruit or veggie

 Multi-grain crackers

 High-fiber granola—eat it dry

 Sunflower or pumpkin seeds

# Winning the battle of the bloat

## WHAT:

It's almost summer, and as the temperature goes up—for many of us—so does our weight. It's not fat we're gaining, though, it's water weight. Does that make you feel better? I didn't think so! Some of us were just born to be bloated. On average, our bodies can carry 6 pounds of extra water a day.

## WHY...
### ...did you get so bloated?

Here are the top three culprits:

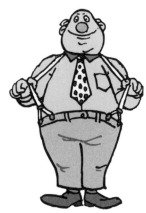

**Alcohol.** Drinking just one or two drinks a day can cause you to become bloated.

**Salt.** An obvious choice, but did you know that most of us eat at least 40 percent more salt daily than our bodies can handle?

**Carbohydrates.** For each gram of carb (breads, cereals) you eat, your body hangs on to two grams of water to help process it. That's why low-carb diets work so well: Cut the carbs and your water weight goes down, and quickly.

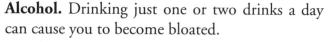

Transform Your Health
in 60 Seconds a Day

# HOW:

There is help, and it doesn't have to come in the form of an over-the-counter drug. It's in the fruit bowl on your kitchen counter. One of the fastest ways to cut bloat is to eat an orange. Citrus is a natural diuretic. It works quickly and the effect lasts for hours.

**Some other easy and healthy ways to beat the bloat:**

 Eat your garnish! Parsley is a natural, mild diuretic.

 Add an extra squeeze of lemon to your iced tea.

 Increase your intake of grapefruit and all types of oranges and tangerines.

 Drink orange or grapefruit juice.

 Squeeze lime juice over salads or stir-fried veggies.

 Eat watermelon—it's also a great natural, mild diuretic.

 Drink more water, which may sound counterproductive, but the more of it you drink, the more you flush out your system.

 Increase exercise. It, too, works as a natural diuretic, flushing water through your system and out through your skin, as sweat.

 For women: Eat and/or take more calcium. Women who don't get enough calcium are more likely to be bloated. Your daily dose should be about 1,200 mg pre-menopause and 1,500 mg post-menopause.

# Beauty foods

## WHAT:

Most of us spend a lot of money each year in pursuit of the perfect shampoo, conditioner, moisturizer and nail polish, ones that will make us look our best. Would you be surprised to learn that even the most expensive products won't work if your diet is poor?

## WHY:

Our hair, skin and nails need certain nutrients and plenty of water to stay healthy and look good.

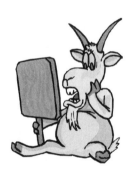

- Healthy hair requires good circulation to the scalp. Poor nutrition results in hair that doesn't grow well or breaks and has split ends. The most commonly lacking healthy-hair nutrients are protein, vitamins B6, B12, C, and folic acid.

- Healthy skin needs all the above nutrients, plus linoleic acid and iron. Without these, your skin may be dry and lifeless.

- Strong nails need protein, selenium, zinc and vitamins C, E and K.

Transform Your Health
in 60 Seconds a Day

# HOW...

# ...to make your hair shiny, your skin radiant, and your nails strong:

**Hair:**

Include lean animal proteins and more lentils and beans, along with at least eight glasses of water daily. Eat fruits with high vitamin C content, such as oranges, grapefruit, kiwis and berries.

**Skin:**

Increase your intake of all fruits, whole-grain products, veggies and lean protein. Be sure to include at least one serving a day of a vitamin A-rich fruit or veggie, since this vitamin is important for maintaining skin moisture and balance. Orange and yellow fruits and veggies are high in vitamin A.

**Hair and Skin:**

In addition to the above, you'll also want to add more essential fatty acids to your diet, since they help keep your skin and hair from becoming dry. Good sources are nuts, seeds, avocados and salmon.

**Nails:**

Include lean protein, either from animal or veggie sources (tofu, beans, lentils), and whole grains. You will also want to include plenty of summer fruits (berries, melons, tropical fruits, peaches, nectarines). Add a smoothie made with blueberries or strawberries and low-fat yogurt (for protein) to your daily routine.

Long-term iron deficiency can lead to brittle, thin and/or spoon-shaped nails, as well as hair loss and itchy skin. The body absorbs iron from red meat more easily than from plant sources, so consider a serving or two of red meat each week. A serving size is 3 ounces, about the size of a deck of cards.

# Vitamin D, the new excuse to sunbathe

## WHAT:

Vitamin D has really been in the news. The latest research has shown that it can help prevent diseases such as cancer and multiple sclerosis (Hayes 2000). In the past few years, researchers have started to pay attention to where most cancers occur geographically. What they've discovered is that more cancers appear in areas where winter months are longer, colder and darker. Additionally, death rates from various cancers, including reproductive system and gastrointestinal cancers, are twice as high in New England when compared to warm and sunny regions like the Southwest.

> If you're wearing sunscreen, your body can't take in enough sun to make vitamin D, so you can occasionally forgo the sunscreen for short periods of time, but keep it nearby and apply it after a few minutes of sun exposure.

## WHY:

Some daily sun exposure is important to help increase your vitamin D levels, but a little goes a long way. Fifteen minutes on a small area of skin, like your arms, can be enough to give your body a good amount of vitamin D.

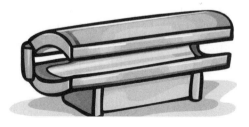

Transform Your Health
in 60 Seconds a Day

# HOW:

After you've enjoyed your 15 minutes of sunning without sunscreen, it's time to practice "safe sun." Here are a few suggestions to protect your skin.

 **Apply early and often.** It takes approximately 20–30 minutes for most sunscreens to absorb into your skin, so make sure you allow ample time for absorption. It's also important to re-apply sunscreen after swimming or sweating. Most sunscreen will protect you for 2–3 hours, so re-apply regularly.

 **Use more rather than less**. Most people use sunscreen too sparingly and don't get the protection they think they are getting. According to most skin-care experts, it takes almost a full ounce (the size of a shot glass) to cover your entire body.

 **Don't forget your ears.** Most of us forget a few important areas while applying sunscreen. These include ears, backs of knees, hands and the tops of your feet.

 **Avoid tanning beds**. There was a rumor circulating years ago that tanning indoors was safer than tanning in the sun. Not true! People who tan at tanning salons have a 2.5 times higher risk of skin cancer.

 **Beware of sunscreens in make-up**. Many cosmetics companies have added sunscreens to foundations and powders. Unfortunately, these stay on your skin for only one to two hours. As your face moves and perspires during the day, the sunscreen will move toward your neck and hairline. So halfway through the day you have little or no protection from the sun.

# Section 5:
# Disease Prevention

# Section 5: Disease Prevention

My new client Tom wanted to lose the 60 pounds he'd gained over the past ten years. Before I started recommending any changes, I suggested he get some basic testing done, including blood pressure, cholesterol and blood glucose levels. He called me in a panic when he got the results—his cholesterol level was a frog's hair under 400, and that, combined with his family history of heart disease, prompted his doctor to tell him he was a time bomb waiting to explode and that if he didn't do something right away to change his lifestyle he was as good as finished. (Note to doctors: Good bedside manner can go a long way here.) Tom asked me to design a cholesterol-lowering, heart-healthy nutrition program for him, along with an exercise routine, and I quickly obliged.

Tom really attacked his new program. He cut his saturated fats and increased his fruits, veggies and whole grains. He also started walking five days a week and added in some weight training. In the first month he lost almost 10 pounds and added a lot of muscle to his frame. He was obviously committed to making permanent changes so that he could sidestep his genetic history. Then he got another call from his doctor. There had been an unfortunate mix-up at the lab, and Tom's cholesterol was really only a little over 200, not the 390 they had originally thought. I never heard from Tom again.

Why do we need a health crisis before we make any permanent changes? I know this is human nature, but if you can stop the train before it derails, putting it back together is much easier.

In this chapter you will find lots of information about common health issues, from constipation and why it can be bad for your health, to how to ease depression by changing your diet, to laughing your way to better health. Laughing does great things for your immune system and circulation, and it helps you sleep like a baby. So next time you see a movie, you might want to make it a comedy.

Transform Your Health
in 60 Seconds a Day

# Fiber—nature's Drāno

## WHAT:

Breast, prostate and other cancers; diabetes; problems with weight loss; high cholesterol; heart disease; diverticulitis; ulcers; constipation—all of these are health problems that can be eased, or possibly prevented, by eating a daily dose of fiber. Hard to believe, isn't it? Just by eating the recommended 25–30 grams of fiber a day, we could all enjoy better health, help prevent disease and lose or maintain weight.

## WHY:

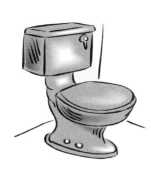

It's a delicate subject, so here is the quick version: Stool is waste, containing all kinds of elements that could potentially cause you harm. The key is to get it out of your body as quickly as possible, and this is where the problems begin. If you're not eating adequate fiber, processing your food can take days. In countries where people do eat ample fiber, the average **transit time** (yes, that's the technical term) is less than *one day.* An American eating the typical American diet may be lucky to have a transit time of *three days.* Someone who is not eating much fiber can take *10 days,* and the elderly can take up to *two weeks.*

But, if you eat enough fiber on a daily basis, you will move things quickly through your system. Your body will be healthier and you will feel much better.

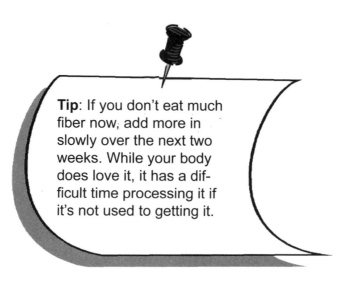

**Tip**: If you don't eat much fiber now, add more in slowly over the next two weeks. While your body does love it, it has a difficult time processing it if it's not used to getting it.

# HOW:

One of the best ways to get fiber is to increase your intake of fresh fruits and veggies and whole grains. Fruits and veggies are especially good because of their high water content, which helps things move along very quickly. Your colon craves water to help process foods.

High-fiber fruits (aim for three or four servings a day):

| | |
|---|---|
| Apple | 3 grams |
| Banana | 2 grams |
| Blueberries (½ cup) | 2 grams |
| Orange | 3 grams |
| Peach | 1.3 grams |
| Pear | 4 grams |
| Raspberries (½ cup) | 6.8 grams |
| Strawberries (½ cup) | 3.8 grams |

Transform Your Health
in 60 Seconds a Day

High-fiber veggies (aim for three or more servings a day):

| | |
|---|---|
| Raw carrots (1 cup) | 4 grams |
| Cooked broccoli (1 cup) | 4.5 grams |
| Raw spinach (2 cups) | 3 grams |
| Cooked cauliflower (1 cup) | 3 grams |
| Sweet potato | 4 grams |
| Peas (½ cup) | 4 grams |

High-fiber whole-grain products (aim for six to eleven servings a day):

| | |
|---|---|
| Whole-grain bread (slice) | 2–3 grams |
| Cooked lentils (1 cup) | 15.6 grams |
| Beans—pinto, black, etc. (½ cup) | 6–7 grams |
| Cooked oatmeal (1 cup) | 3 grams |
| Brown rice (1 cup) | 4 grams |

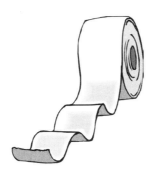

# Brain food: eating intelligently

## WHAT:

We know that what we eat can impact our cancer and heart disease risk. New research is showing us that food can affect how our brains function too, for both the short and long term. Foods high in essential fatty acids (EFAs), folic acid (FA) and antioxidants are topping the list of "must-haves" for healthy brains. EFAs must be obtained through diet. They are called "essential" because the body can't make them.

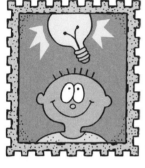

## WHY:

**EFAs** (also known as omega-3 fatty acids) may help prevent Alzheimer's disease and dementia, depression and ADD/HD. According to National Institutes of Health researcher Norman Salem, Jr., "Populations that consume large amounts of fish have much lower rates of major depression." (Stoll 1995). Your brain is more than 60 percent fat. It functions best when it gets a constant supply of healthy fats. Over 2,000 studies document the benefits of eating fish (or supplementing with fish oils).

We also now know that diets lacking in EFAs can result in these other health challenges: weight gain or great difficulty losing weight, swollen joints (due to the lack of anti-inflammatory effect of EFAs), lack of concentration (due to a lack of essential brain fat), arthritis, weight loss, macular degeneration, cardiovascular disease, behavior or

Transform Your Health
in 60 Seconds a Day

aggression problems, sleeping problems, mood swings, dry skin, eczema, poor circulation, fatigue and immune system weakness.

**Folic acid** deficiency, which is very common in the U.S., can cause psychiatric disorders, notably depression. Further, when your brain level of FA is low, serotonin, the body's feel-good chemical, will plummet.

**Antioxidants** help keep your body and brain from aging. Oxygen will age you from the inside out, so you need a huge dose of *anti*oxidants to balance this impact.

---

**Interesting fact:** Until the 1950s, the main canned fish people ate was sardines, one of the best sources of miraculous EFAs. When food manufacturers switched from canning sardines to canning tuna (from which most of the fat is removed), rates of depression began to rise. At the same time, we were seeing the emergence of processed foods. So the food that Americans began buying was now low in fiber, high in sugar and salt, and low in essential fatty acids—a recipe for depression and other health problems.

---

# HOW...

## ...to boost your brain function by eating smart:

 **Essential Fatty Acids\*:** Healthy fats are abundant in fatty fish such as salmon, trout and sardines. *A word of caution:* While eating more wild fish is helpful, eating farmed fish is not. Farmed fish have higher levels of pesticides than wild fish, but wild fish can also be contaminated. Purified fish oils may be the answer. When it comes to purchasing fish oils you get what you pay for. The more expensive brands are usually cleaner, with pesticides and other contaminants removed.

### How much a day?

Most of us would benefit by eating at least two sources of good fat daily.

 **Folic Acid:** The words folate and folic acid come from the word foliage, which means leafage. Spinach, broccoli and peas are great sources of FA. But most of us cook these foods before we eat them, and that can destroy *almost half* their FA content. It's very important to get FA from a variety of food sources, some of them raw. Beyond green leafy veggies, oranges, bananas, grapefruit and strawberries are a great way to up your intake. So are grain products, which are now fortified with FA as a result of research that strongly correlated low FA levels with heart disease and birth defects.

### How much a day?

A serving of fortified cereal daily, along with five to six servings of fruits and veggies, will provide the RDA of 400 mcgs per day.

---

\*EFAs are blood thinners, so if you're currently taking a blood thinner check with your physician before supplementing with EFAs.

  Transform Your Health
in 60 Seconds a Day

**Antioxidants:** Blueberries. I've heard some nutritionists call them brain berries! According to Steven Pratt M.D., author of the book "SuperFoods Rx: Fourteen Foods That Will Change Your Life," just one cup of blueberries provides as much antioxidant benefit as five servings of apples, carrots, broccoli or squash. These berries have been shown to reduce age-related conditions such as Alzheimer's disease and dementia.

### How much a day?

Eat a cup a day. While blueberries are best, you can also increase amounts of other similarly colored foods such as purple grapes, blackberries, raspberries, boysenberries, strawberries and cherries. Add a heaping tablespoon of organic blueberry spread to pancakes, yogurt or toast.

Oregano is another great way to give yourself a big antioxidant boost. (See the chapter "Spice up your life" on page 74.)

**Other Powerful Brain Foods:**

 Tomatoes

 Soy Products

 Nuts

 Avocados

 Sunflower and pumpkin seeds

 Flaxseeds—ground or oil (For more about the wonders of flax, see the next chapter "Just give me the flax.")

# Just give me the flax

## WHAT:

Flaxseed has been around for thousands of years (it's even mentioned in the Bible). Why are so many people talking about it now, and can it really help you a live longer, healthier life? In a word, YES!

Flax is helpful in alleviating over 60 health conditions. Some of these are cancer (flaxseed contains at least 27 cancer-preventing compounds), allergies, high blood pressure, acne, eczema, psoriasis, breast pain, immune disorders, vision problems, heart attacks, joint problems, high cholesterol, multiple sclerosis, arthritis, ADD, and depression. Eating flaxseed will even help prevent dandruff and dry, cracking winter skin.

## WHY:

Flaxseed is one of the richest sources of omega-3 fatty acids available. This fatty acid is pivotal to the health of your body and brain (see the chapter "Brain food: eating intelligently" on page 108). The only problem is, it's almost impossible to get enough from food (another rich source is seal blubber; see what I mean?). So you have to supplement your diet to meet your needs.

The other healthy substance in flax is lignans, contained in the outer hull of the seed. Lignans are a rich source of antioxidants, so rich, in fact, that you would need to eat about 100 slices of whole-wheat bread to get the same amount of antioxidants as in two tablespoons of flaxseed.

People stopped eating foods rich in omega-3 fatty acids for many reasons. Let's face it; sardines for dinner don't sound that satisfying, and most of us don't spend much time baking these days. Hundreds of years ago flaxseed was used in all homemade breads and baked goods. One reason we stopped using flax is that the seeds and oil turn rancid quickly. Once it's ground or the package opened, it can spoil in just days.

# HOW...
## ...to add flax to your diet:

Flaxseed comes in three forms—oil, whole seed or ground seed.

**Ground Flax:** The seed must be ground for the nutrients to be released. I purchase it already ground and store it in the freezer. Sprinkle on cereal, salads, sauces (spaghetti is great), chili, soups, scrambled eggs (my favorite) or steamed veggies. Add to pancake or muffin batter and other baked goods.

**Flax Oil:** Oil is a great source, but make sure you store it in the darkest part of your fridge, since flax hates light! Blend with smoothies, yogurt, applesauce, roasted veggies, salad dressings, chili, soup, or drizzle over fish or chicken. Flax oil can't be used in cooking, though—the high heat will destroy all the health benefits—so add it after cooking.

The jury is still out on the amount of oil or seed to consume. Most studies are using one to two tablespoons per day.

# Meet the phytochemicals. No, they're not the latest rock band!

## WHAT:

Phytochemicals are substances similar to vitamins, and they are responsible for giving plants their color and taste. They are found in all plant-based foods, including teas, spices and herbs ("phyto" means plant). We don't know how they work, but they are powerful ammunition in the war against cancer.

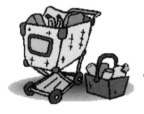

Phytochemicals have been shown to:

- Attack tumors by blocking or reducing their blood supply

- Prevent cell mutations that lead to cancer

- Prevent oxidation (similar to rust) in the cells of the body

- Strengthen the immune system

- Prevent heart disease, diabetes and high blood pressure

## WHY:

The vibrant colors of fruits and veggies all mean something different to your body. I often tell my clients to "eat by color" and try to include two green, one red, one yellow and one purple food in your daily diet.

Transform Your Health
in 60 Seconds a Day

# HOW:

**Red foods** (cancer fighters):

Berries, grapes, red onions, tomatoes, apples, watermelon and cherries

**Blue and purple foods** (cancer fighters and brain health):

Blueberries, blackberries, raisins, eggplant, purple cabbage, plums and prunes

**Green foods** (cancer fighters and eye health):

Asparagus, broccoli, green cabbage, avocados, parsley (and other any green herb), spinach and green beans

**White, yellow and orange foods** (heart health and cancer fighters):

Carrots, corn, lemons, apricots, yellow onions, garlic, bananas, mangos, pineapples and oranges

**Interesting tidbit:** One orange has over 170 different phytochemicals that can inhibit tumor growth and bloods clots.

See the chapter "French fries are not veggies" on page 64 for ideas on sneaking fruits and veggies into your diet.

# Why your cholesterol counts

## WHAT:

Cholesterol is present in all of us, and our bodies make enough of it to be able to carry out certain essential functions, including the creation of hormones, bile acid, and vitamin D. Cholesterol enters your body in two ways—you make it in your liver and you ingest it in your food.

Elevated levels of blood cholesterol contribute greatly to heart disease. Recently, drug companies have been promoting cholesterol-lowering drugs called statins, and many physicians are prescribing them.

## WHY:

Statins, like most drugs, carry a long list of side effects, including nausea, constipation, diarrhea, memory loss, and muscle pain and wasting.

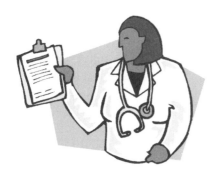

Transform Your Health
in 60 Seconds a Day

# HOW:

A study in the *American Journal of Clinical Nutrition* showed that tofu, almonds, cereal fibers, plant sterols and soy products can lower total cholesterol more effectively than statin drugs (Jenkins and others 2006). Talk to your physician about including these foods in your diet to help lower your cholesterol naturally.

 **Blueberries** can lower cholesterol as much as some statin drugs. They contain a substance called pterostilbene, which activates a cellular structure that lowers cholesterol. Add blueberries to the top of your cereal or yogurt, add frozen ones to your smoothies, or top your toast with all natural blueberry preserves or jam.

 **Almonds** have been shown to decrease cholesterol levels by 14 percent when 3 ounces are eaten daily. Most of the fat in almonds is unsaturated and contains no cholesterol. Almonds are full of folic acid, and folic acid has been shown to lower homocystein (this substance has been shown to cause fatty build-up in arteries). Eat a small handful a day, or try switching to almond butter, instead of peanut butter, on your toast.

 **Garlic.** A Penn State study discovered that substances in garlic can lower cholesterol in the liver by 40–60 percent in laboratory tests (Yeh and Liu 2001). Garlic is truly one of the most nutritious foods nature ever designed. For convenience, buy your garlic already peeled, store in your refrigerator, chop it and add to as many dishes as possible. If your whole family eats it, not only will you all be healthier, you will all be stinky together so no one will complain about your breath.

# The type 2 diabetes disaster

## WHAT:

Type 2 diabetes, the kind most commonly associated with older adults but now seen more in younger adults and even children, and pre-diabetes (abnormal blood sugars) affect 73 million Americans. Diabetes is a chronic disease that results in dangerously high blood sugars. Some of the health risks associated with poorly managed diabetes are heart disease, kidney failure, nerve damage and blindness.

## WHY:

The pancreas makes a hormone called insulin, which is released into the bloodstream in response to a rise in blood sugar that occurs when we eat. It "grabs" blood sugar and escorts it into cells for use later as energy, thereby keeping blood sugars at normal levels. With type 2 diabetes, the body may still make some insulin, but it may not be enough, and the body may not be able to use it properly. Type 2 diabetes is considered a disease of a lifestyle that includes over-consumption of sugar, white-flour and processed foods, coupled with being sedentary and overweight.

Transform Your Health
in 60 Seconds a Day

# HOW...

## ...to prevent diabetes if you don't have it, or help control it if you do*:

 Weight loss and exercise can delay the onset of diabetes in those most likely to develop it. Losing as little as 5 percent of your current body weight (or 10 pounds on average), can reduce diabetes risk by 58 percent. Exercise also appears to make the cells more receptive to insulin, meaning the body is able to use insulin more efficiently.

 A high-fiber diet can prevent a rapid rise in blood sugar, helping control or prevent this disease. (See the chapter "Fiber—nature's Drāno" on page 105 for ways to increase your daily fiber intake.)

 Add cinnamon to your diet! A half teaspoon a day can significantly reduce blood sugar levels in those with type 2 diabetes. It also reduces triglyceride levels, LDL (bad cholesterol) and total cholesterol levels. Sprinkle a little cinnamon on fresh fruit and yogurt, or break up a cinnamon stick and place it in your coffee maker with the grounds.

---

*Type 2 diabetes is a serious medical condition that requires professional medical care. These recommendations are intended as informational only and should not be substituted for medical care. If you have type 2 diabetes, you may want to discuss this information with your health care team to see if it fits into your management plan.

# Laugh your way to health

## WHAT:

Are you happy? Are you surprised that I care? While you may think it an odd question, being happy can be a huge boost to your health. People who are happy have stronger immune systems, lower cholesterol levels and clearer arteries, *and that's just for starters!* One study on the effects of happiness followed people from birth to death and found that the happy optimists lived longer (much longer) and had fewer cancers, heart disease, and other life-threatening diseases than the pessimists (van Doorn 1999).

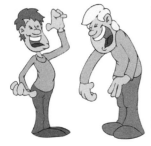

## WHY:

Laughing helps release endorphins, the feel-good chemical that evens out our moods and makes us happy and relaxed. Have you ever had problems trying to lose weight? Would you be surprised to learn that happiness can greatly affect your ability to do so? Studies have shown that women who experience high levels of stress (these are not happy women) have a more difficult time losing weight (Kivimäki and others 2006). These women also have lower energy levels and are often depressed. The good news is that laughing can help diffuse stress and increase your energy levels, allowing your body to relax and start to lose weight.

Transform Your Health
in 60 Seconds a Day

# HOW...
# ...laughing improves health:

☺   Increases immunity, helping us fight off colds and diseases such as cancer and heart disease.

☺   Increases endorphin levels, keeping our moods steady. In fact, the endorphins released from one minute of laughing are equal to that released from 10 minutes of strenuous rowing.

☺   Increases energy. Have you ever had uncontrollable giggles when you were really tired? Laughing is our body's way to increase your energy level.

☺   Keeps our arteries clear and cholesterol levels lower.

☺   Relaxes all of our muscles and decreases muscle tension.

We're so busy scheduling appointments that we forget to take a moment and just laugh. A good laugh can dramatically change our brain chemistry; our body feels better and our cells function more effectively. Happiness doesn't usually just happen—we have to work on creating it.

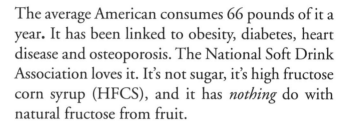

# Sweet and innocent?

## WHAT:

The average American consumes 66 pounds of it a year. It has been linked to obesity, diabetes, heart disease and osteoporosis. The National Soft Drink Association loves it. It's not sugar, it's high fructose corn syrup (HFCS), and it has *nothing* do with natural fructose from fruit.

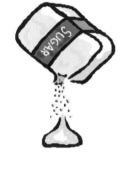

In 1966, sucrose (table sugar) was the most popular sugar in use. Today, HFCS is the No. 1 sweetener used in products ranging from sodas (13 teaspoons per 12-ounce can) to jams, jellies and even ketchup (one-third of it is HFCS). Food manufacturers love it because it's very sweet and very cheap. Farmers love it because it comes from corn, providing a market for the common glut of corn crops. It's almost impossible to find a processed-food product without HFCS. Not only does it make food sweeter, it also extends the shelf life of many products and prevents freezer burn.

## WHY:

Have you ever heard the expression: "You can't fool Mother Nature"? HFCS is an example of just that. When your body consumes HFCS it doesn't process it the same way it does regular table sugar or naturally occurring sugars in fruit. When consuming "real" sugar, your body produces hormones that turn down appetite and fat storage, and you produce another hormone that turns off hunger pangs so you won't overeat. When you consume

Transform Your Health
in 60 Seconds a Day

HFCS, none of these hormones are produced, so in the long run you could gain weight because you never feel full when consuming HFCS.

# HOW...
## ...to cut the HFCS out of your diet:

Become an avid label reader and check for HFCS. Avoid foods that contain it whenever possible.

Eat more fruit if you need to satisfy a sweet tooth.

Try natural sweeteners such as xylitol and stevia. Both can be used in coffee, tea and baking. (See the next chapter, "Some sweet alternatives.")

# Some sweet alternatives

## WHAT:

Xylitol and stevia are two safe sweeteners that are made from natural substances.

**Xylitol** has many names, including wood sugar or birch sugar. It's made from natural substances, including birch, raspberries and plums. Created by a German chemist in the late 1800s, it rose in popularity during World War II, when sugar was scarce. It's a sugar alcohol and at high doses may cause some mild stomach distress. (Yes, that's the politically correct term for diarrhea.) It has been studied extensively at high doses, and it appears to cause no other adverse health effects in humans. Xylitol looks like sugar and tastes like sugar but has 40 percent fewer calories than table sugar. Since the 1960s it has been used as the preferred sweetener for diabetics in Russia, Germany, Japan and Switzerland.

**Stevia** is a plant that is almost 300 times sweeter than table sugar. It has a negligible effect on blood sugar (it's almost calorie-free), so it's attractive to diabetics and others on carbohy-drate-controlled diets.

## WHY:

No health risks are associated with either of these sweeteners, and xylitol even has some health benefits. It reduces tooth decay (by replacing other dietary sugars), and recent research confirms that it has a plaque-reducing effect and that it may even help repair teeth that have been damaged by cavities (Tanzer 1995). This is why xylitol is so commonly used in sugar-free gum.

## HOW:

Both of these sweeteners come in crystalline sugar form, so they resemble table sugar. Both can be used in baking, but stevia does have a slight aftertaste, so it may take a little while to get used to it.

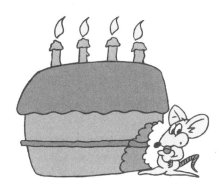

# Green tea gets the green light

## WHAT:

The most highly consumed beverage in the world is water. No. 2 is tea. Tea is full of health-producing, disease-reducing, anti-aging antioxidants. The Chinese have known about the health benefits of green tea since ancient times, using it to treat ailments such as headaches, stomach disorders and depression, to name just a few. Cultures that drink primarily tea compared to cultures that drink primarily sweetened drinks have much lower levels of disease.

## WHY:

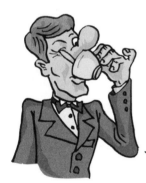

One cup of green tea provides 10–40 mg of polyphenols (antioxidants), and the health effects are greater than a serving of broccoli, spinach, carrots or strawberries. The high antioxidant activity of green tea protects the body from oxidative damage due to free radicals.

Drinking green tea has also been shown to:

- Increase bone density

- Lower risk of cavities by 75 percent

- Help prevent kidney stones

- Decrease the risk of breast, prostate, pancreatic, colorectal, esophageal, bladder and lung cancer

Lower the risk of heart attack and stroke

# HOW:

 Drink high quality, organic green tea. Researchers are still trying to determine how much to drink for good health. Most recommend two or three cups a day.

 Green tea does have caffeine, although much lower levels than black tea or coffee. Your body assimilates the caffeine in green tea differently than caffeine from black tea or coffee, so you won't feel the same kind of caffeine "high" or "low" that you might feel from coffee.

 Decaffeinated green tea has fewer health benefits than regular green tea, depending on the process used. Look for green tea that is decaffeinated using the effervescence method, which retains 95 percent of the antioxidants. The other decaffeinating process, which uses solvents, retains only 30 percent of the antioxidants.

 Make your own decaf! Eighty percent of the caffeine is released in the first 45 seconds of steeping, so just dump your cup after a minute or less of steeping, refill it with hot water, use the same tea bag, and you will have a very natural version of "almost" decaffeinated tea.

 Squeeze your tea bag! According to Steven Pratt, M.D., author of "SuperFoods Rx: Fourteen Foods That Will Change Your Life," squeezing the last bit of tea from your bag doubles the antioxidant amount you get (p. 159).

# The high cost of being overweight

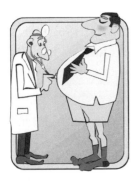

## WHAT:

We are a nation of chronically overweight people. In fact, 61 percent of Americans are either overweight or obese. Between 1991 and 2002, the percentage of overweight Americans more than doubled.

## WHY:

It's easy to see how this happened:

 Computers have made us very sedentary.

 Commuting to work keeps us sitting for hours on end.

 Restaurants have "super-sized" food portions so that one order now buys more food for less money, and most of us eat everything we see on our plate. (For more about super-sizing, see the chapter "How big is your bagel?" on page 14.)

 We work longer hours and have less play time (calorie-burning time) than ever before.

Transform Your Health
in 60 Seconds a Day

But did you know that just an extra 100 calories a day could put 10 pounds of fat on your frame each year?

Overweight people are at higher risk of type 2 diabetes, heart disease, arthritis, gout and most types of cancers. They are also at much higher risk of dying in car accidents that healthy-weight people survive. Most of us know it doesn't take much to be overweight and unhealthy. An extra 100 calories is simple to add to your daily diet. How many times in the last week have you grabbed a handful of potato chips or had the whipped cream on your coffee drink? These habits are each worth 100 calories or more!

The professional costs of being overweight are similar to the personal costs, plus employees over their healthy weight are absent more often, produce less work and cost their employers about $500 more per year in health care costs. Compare these figures from a study reported in 1998 (Burton and others 1998):

$ A healthy-weight employee costs approximately $114 in health care per year.

$ An overweight employee costs approximately $513 in health care per year.

$ An obese employee costs approximately $620 in health care per year.

# HOW...

## ...to cut back on those extra 100 calories a day and begin the process of healthy weight loss and improved energy and longevity:

 Never eat leftovers off anyone's plate. This can easily save you 100–300 calories a day.

 Cut out all sodas. This will save you at least 200 calories a day. Also, the sugar in soda just serves to increase your appetite, causing you to eat more later.

 Order salads with the dressing on the side, and dress lightly. Most Americans get 60–70 percent of their fat calories each day from the dressing.

 Order the non-cream based soup instead of the salad. Often the soup will have more nutritional value than the salad and will also serve to depress your appetite.

Transform Your Health
in 60 Seconds a Day

# Section 6:
## Stress

# Section 6: Stress

Sharon burned the candle at both ends. She worked full time, had two teenage boys, had a husband who traveled at least three days a week, and recently started taking care of her elderly parents. She was obviously stressed, tired and overwhelmed. She was also carrying 75 extra pounds. Weight was something she had always struggled with. Sharon came to see me for some ideas about how to eat well on the run so she could maintain her fast-paced lifestyle.

I could have designed the best weight-loss program in the world for Sharon, but if she didn't deal with her chronic stress, her body would look at each meal as an opportunity to add fat to her thighs. Add to this the fact that Sharon wasn't sleeping much, another set-up for weight gain. This sleep deprivation was also making it hard for her body to heal areas that needed to be healed, add new bone or grow her hair.

Initially Sharon didn't want to discuss her stress levels, she just wanted a quick food plan so she could be on her way (sound familiar?) But she soon realized that, while eating healthier food would help, if she didn't find ways to manage her stress she was at risk for many stress-related diseases such as heart disease, stroke and diabetes. Once Sharon began taking better care of herself physically and emotionally—walking at lunch, getting into bed a half-hour earlier at night, scheduling regular fun time out with friends and co-workers (something she hadn't done in years)— she felt much more in control and upbeat, and she lost 50 pounds in the process!

Stressful situations and the stressors of fast-paced lifestyles can harm us in many ways, some of them surprising and seemingly unrelated. This chapter may help you alter your lifestyle by giving you insight into the many ways stress can affect your health.

# I can't find my keys! Stress and its effects on your body and brain

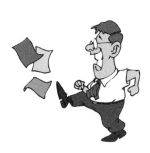

## WHAT:

Everyone experiences stress. Some stress is good for us because it compels us to get more projects done at work or home. But these days, stress is at an all-time high and our bodies and minds don't respond to it quite the same. Some of us experience out-of-control appetite, headaches, nausea, depression, burnout and a depressed immune system, resulting in a big bad cold.

## WHY:

**...do I get sick every time I get stressed out?**

When stressed, our body increases its production of stress chemicals to help us fight off the stress. This is the typical "fight-or-flight" response. These stress hormones can attack your immune system, making it an easy target for germs and bugs.

**...does being under stress kill my energy?**

High levels of stress can wreak havoc with your blood flow, leaving your energy center (your brain) undernourished.

**...is my hair falling out?**

The ongoing release of stress hormones during times of chronic stress can cause a slowdown in hair growth, and eventually your hair will start to thin and fall out.

### ...can't I remember where I left my keys?

Chronic stress can shrink the area of your brain that is in charge of memory and learning, causing these very important brain cells to die off.

### ...is my heartburn driving me crazy?

Stress causes stomach acid to be produced at high levels and digestive enzymes to be produced at low levels. The combination of these factors makes your body more prone to heartburn, acid reflux and ulcers. Take a look at the life of stressed-out air traffic controllers—those working at high-stress airports in Chicago and New York have almost twice the incidence of gastrointestinal upset as do controllers working in less stressful airports in Virginia and Ohio.

Transform Your Health
in 60 Seconds a Day

# HOW...

## ... to curb stress naturally (you can't always control stress, but you can change your reaction to it):

🌹     Apply a cold compress to the back of your neck for about 10 minutes. This will help increase energy flow to the brain and boost the effect of the feel-good hormone serotonin, which will help calm you down.

🌹     Include more pineapple in your diet during stressful times. Pineapple contains bromelain, which can act as a stomach enzyme and help ease the problems of digestion.

🌹     Drink ginger tea or chew on ginger candy. Ginger has been shown to soothe stomach irritation, inflammation and nausea.

🌹     Go outside. This is my personal favorite. Being outside can change your reactions, fast. If you can't get outside, go to the bathroom and get some quiet time.

🌹     Surround yourself with pictures that make you smile. Studies have shown that your brain can't hold two conflicting thoughts at the same time, so if you are feeling angry, look at a picture of someone who makes you laugh—your brain will latch onto the new and more pleasant thought.

🌹     Exercise more often. Exercise can turn your body into a fortress against stress by reducing its negative reactions to stress.

🌹     Invest in some music or audio books for your commute. Shifting your focus from traffic to something you enjoy can make it much easier to change your thoughts from negative to positive.

🌹     Breathe better. When stressed, the first place to be hit is our respiratory system. Our breathing gets shallow and sometimes rapid. To be a better breather, practice belly breathing: Place one hand on your stomach; on the inhale, the stomach goes out; on the exhale, it flattens. Within seconds of breathing like this you will lower your blood pressure, slow your heart rate and stop the stress-reaction cycle.

# Got stress? Got fat?

## WHAT:

You already know that stress can make you feel frazzled, out of control and anxious, and it can shorten your life by helping speed up the process of diseases such as high blood pressure and diabetes. *But did you know that stress can also make you fat? And that it can keep you fat?* It's now a scientific fact: Your stress levels, and how you handle stress, can determine your fat level, overall health and even your appetite.

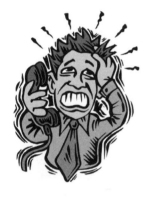

## WHY:

Your body can handle a good amount of stress, but it wasn't built to withstand chronic stress. We were designed to survive using the fight-or-flight system—we either took on the stressor (we fought the saber tooth tiger), or we ran from it. With either response, there was physical movement on our part, and that's what is missing today in our response to stress.

Our bodies react to stress by creating stress hormones. These hormones encourage the following responses:

- Blood pressure, and heart and breathing rates increase.

- Blood moves from internal organs to the legs (so you can run).

Transform Your Health
in 60 Seconds a Day

- Digestion, pain and immune system responses are put on hold.

How stress makes you fat:

When stressed, your appetite is temporarily turned off. When the stress subsides, your body tries to return to normal, but the stress hormones have other ideas. These hormones stay elevated so that you will crave carbs (sugar) and fat, assuring that you will replace the calories burned during the last stress response to prepare for the next one. Though modern day stressors don't usually require you to burn extraordinary amounts of calories, your body's reaction to stress has not changed, so you still load up on carbs and fats after stressful incidents, and you store these extra calories as fat. And guess where you store this wonderful "stress fat"? Right in your stomach, so it's close to all of your internal organs, which makes for easy deployment during episodes of stress.

# HOW...

## ...to turn your body into a fortress against "stress fat":

Research has shown that one of the most effective protections from stress is consistent exercise. Exercise gives your stress hormones a job to do. When "busy," these hormones are less likely to store fat in your stomach area. You don't need to do a long, hard workout routine, but you do need to be consistent.

- After a stressful incident, take a five- to 10-minute walk.

- Find an excuse to take the stairs or walk over to see a friend for a few minutes. Climbing stairs is very helpful in diffusing stress.

- Walk for 30 minutes, three times a week, to help prevent stress fat from lodging in your stomach.

- Practice yoga, Pilates and strength training to really protect your body from the harmful physical health effects of stress as well as stress fat.

Transform Your Health
in 60 Seconds a Day

# When the going gets tough, why men go into their caves and women go to lunch

## WHAT:

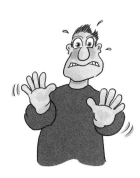

Men and women are vastly different in what stresses them out and how they handle it. Women stress about multiple things—since we are so good at multi-tasking, we are apparently good at multi-stressing too. Men, on the other hand, appear to stress about one thing at a time. According to psychologist Carl Pickhardt Ph.D., a psychologist, spokesman for the American Psychological Association and author of *The Everything Parent's Guide to Positive Discipline,* men and women enter into the stress cycle very differently and for different reasons. Men get stressed when they feel their performance is at risk or will be judged. Women enter the stress cycle when their relationships are threatened, when they feel pressured to take on a project they really don't have time for, and when they don't have enough time for self-care.

So while a woman gets up in the morning and stresses about making breakfast, getting the kids to school on time, getting herself to work on time, finishing that proposal, planning what the family will have for dinner and how she's going to get her workout in, her husband is stressing about one or two things, perhaps a meeting with his accountant or a business presentation at lunch.

When stressed, men tend to want to escape into their caves for some quiet time, while women have a desire to nurture and socialize with others, or "tend and befriend," as reported in *Psychological Review* (Taylor and others 2000).

## WHY:

One word: HORMONES! You can blame it all on a hormone called oxytocin. Women secrete more of this hormone, and once combined with other female hormones, it creates the tend and befriend response. Men secrete less, which leads to the fight-or-flight response.

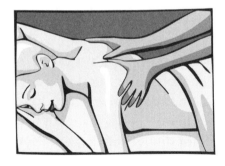

Transform Your Health
in 60 Seconds a Day

# HOW...
## ...to deal with stress:

 Women, don't get mad at your husband for his lack of multi-task stressing; he just isn't wired to do that. The best way to manage your stress (besides saying no to projects or people that over-demand your dwindling time) is to stay connected and social. If you can talk to someone about your challenges, and do it while enjoying something physical such as walking, or even shopping (yes, I'm suggesting retail therapy), then you can manage your stress with fewer negative physical effects.

 Men, your best bet is to focus on an escape. Go into your cave, alone, or do something active like playing golf. It's competitive and physical—a perfect combination for combating male stress.

# References

Ahn, Juhee and I. U. Grün. 2005. "Heterocyclic amines: Inhibitory effects of natural extracts on the formation of polar and nonpolar heterocyclic amines in cooked beef." *Journal of Food Science* 70 (4): C263–C268.

Bazzano, Lydia A., J. He, L. G. Ogden, C. Loria, S. Vupputuri, L. Myers and P. K. Whelton. 2001. "Legume consumption and risk of coronary heart disease in US men and women: NHANES I Epidemiologic follow-up study." *Archives of Internal Medicine* 161:2573–2578.

Brown, Melody, et al. 2004. "Carotenoid bioavailability is higher from salads ingested with full-fat than with fat-reduced salad dressings as measured with electrochemical detection." *American Journal of Clinical Nutrition* 80:396–403.

Burton, W.N., C.Y. Chen, A.B. Schultz, D.W. Edington. 1998. "The economic costs associated with body mass index in a workplace." *Journal of Occupational and Environmental Medicine* 40 (9): 786–792.

Chiavacci, Anne. 2002. "Dietary fats ... friend or foe?" Published on dietary fats page of www.intelihealth.com. Accessed October 2006.

Enstrom, James E. 2001. www.vitalnutrients.net. Accessed June 2003.

The Environmental Working Group. 2006. www.ewg.org. From "What's the difference?" Web page (from Organic food standards, to Shopper's guide, to What's the difference? page). Accessed October 2006.

Fazekas, Zsuzsanna, D. Gao, R. N. Saladi, Y. Lu and M. Lebwohl, H. 2003. "Protective effects of lycopene against ultraviolet B-induced photodamage." *Nutrition and Cancer* 47(2): 181–7.

Greenwald, Peter, Director of the Division of Cancer Prevention, National Cancer Institute. 2002. www.cancer.gov/ncicancerbulletin/ NCI. Accessed September 2005.

Hattori A, Migitaka H, Iigo M, et al. 1995. "Identification of melatonin in plants and its effects on plasma melatonin levels and binding to melatonin receptors in vertebrates." *Biochemistry and Molecular Biology International* 35 (3): 627–34.

Hayes, C.E. 2000. "Vitamin D: A natural inhibitor of multiple sclerosis." *The Proceedings of the Nutrition Society* 59 (4): 531–5.

Jenkins, David, C. W. Kendall, D. A. Faulkner, et al. 2006. "Assessment of the longer-term effects of a dietary portfolio of cholesterol-lowering foods in hypercholesterolemia." *American Journal of Clinical Nutrition* 83 (3): 582-91.

Khan, Alam, M. Safdar, M. Khan, K. Khattak and R. Anderson. 2003. "Cinnamon improves glucose and lipids of people with type 2 diabetes." *Diabetes Care* 26:3215–3218.

Kivimäki, Mika, J. Head, J. E. Ferrie, M. J. Shipley, E. Brunner, J. Vahtera and M. G. Marmot. 2006. "Work stress, weight gain and weight loss: Evidence for bidirectional effects of job strain on body mass index in the Whitehall II study." *International Journal of Obesity* 30:982–987.

Levine, James and N. Eberhardt. 1999. "The role of nonexercise activity in thermogenesis in resistance to fat gain in humans." *Science* 283:212–214.

Mancini-Filho, J., A. Van-Koiij, D. A. Mancini, F.F. Cozzolino and R. P. Torres. 1998. "Antioxidant activity of cinnamon (Cinnamomum Zeylanicum, Breyne) extracts." *Bollettino chimico farmaceutico* 137 (11): 443–7.

Transform your health
60 seconds at a time

Mattes, Richard. 1999. "Effects of chronic peanut consumption on energy balance and hedonics." *International Journal of Obesity* 26 (August): 1129–37.

Mattes, Richard and S.K. Voisard. "Effects of Peanuts on Hunger and Food Intakes in Humans." Presentation, Experimental Biology '98. April 20, 1998, Pittsburgh, Pennsylvania.

Nerurkar P.V., L. Le Marchand and R.V. Cooney. 1999. "Effects of marinating with Asian marinades or western barbecue sauce on PhIP and MeIQx formation in barbecued beef." *Nutrition and Cancer* 34 (2): 147–52.

Pattison, D.J., A.J. Silman and N.J. Goodson. 2004. "Vitamin C and the risk of developing inflammatory polyarthritis: Prospective nested case-control study." *Annals of the Rheumatic Diseases* 63 (July): 843–847.

Pickhardt, Carl. 2003. *The Everything Parent's Guide to Positive Discipline: Professional Advice for Raising a Well-behaved Child.* Avon, Massachusetts: Adams Media, 2003.

Pizzorno Jr., Joseph and M. T. Murray. 1999. *Textbook of Natural Medicine, 2nd ed.*, 1111–1116. New York: Churchill Livingstone Publishing, 1999.

Pratt, S. and K. Matthews. 2004. *SuperFoods Rx: Fourteen Foods that Will Change Your Life.* New York: HarperCollins, 2004.

Schabath, Matthew and S. Spitz. 2006. "Phytoestrogens and risk of lung cancer—Reply." *Journal of the American Medical Association.* 295:755–756

Stahl, Wilhelm, U. Heinrich, H. Jungmann, H. Sies, and H. Tronnier. 2000. "Carotenoids and carotenoids plus vitamin E protect against ultraviolet light-induced erythema in humans." *American Journal of Clinical Nutrition* 71 (March): 795–798.

Stoll, Andrew L., et al. 1995. "Omega 3 fatty acids in bipolar disorder." *American Journal of Clinical Nutrition* 62 (July): 1-9.

Tanzer, JM.1995. "Xylitol chewing gum and dental caries." *International Dental Journal* 45 (Suppl 1): 65–76.

Taylor, S.E., L.C. Klein, B.P. Lewis, and T.L. Gruenewald. 2000. "Biobehavioral responses to stress in females: Tend-and-befriend, not fight-or-flight." *Psychological Review* 107 (3): 411–429.

Van Doorn, Carol. 1999. "A qualitative approach to studying health optimism, realism, and pessimism." *Research on Aging* 21 (3): 440–457

Vander Wal et al. 2005. "Short-term effect of eggs on satiety in overweight and obese subjects." *Journal of the American College of Nutrition* 24:510–515.

Weil, Andrew. 2002. "Aspartame, can a little bit hurt?" On www.drweil.com. Accessed in November 2006.

Welsh, Jean A., M. E. Cogswell, S. Rogers, H. Rockett, Z. Mei, and L. M. Grummer-Strawn. 2005. "Overweight among low-income preschool children associated with the consumption of sweet drinks: Missouri, 1999–2002." *Pediatrics* 115 (February): e223–e229.

Yeh, Y.Y. and L. Liu. 2001. "Cholesterol-lowering effect of garlic extracts and organosulfur compounds: Human and animal studies." *Journal of Nutrition* 131:989s-993s.

Transform your health
60 seconds at a time